MEDICAL UTOPIAS

ETHICAL PERSPECTIVES MONOGRAPH SERIES

4

Medical Utopias
Ethical Reflections about Emerging Medical Technologies

Bert Gordijn

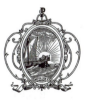

PEETERS

LEUVEN – PARIS – DUDLEY, MA

2006

Library of Congress Cataloging-in-Publication Data

Gordijn, Bert, 1965-
   [Medizinische Utopien. English]
   Medical utopias : ethical reflections about emerging medical technologies / Bert
   Gordijn.
      p. cm. -- (Ethical perspectives monograph series)
   Includes bibliographical references.
   ISBN 90-429-1700-8 (alk. paper)
      1. Medical ethics. 2. Bioethics. 3. Utopias. I. Title. II. Series.

   R724G679513 2005
   174.2--dc22

                                                            2005054739

Translated into English by Sarah L Kirkby

ISBN-10   90-429-1700-8
ISBN-13   9789042917002
D. 2006/0602/3

© 2006, Peeters – Bondgenotenlaan 153 – B-3000 Leuven – Belgium

TABLE OF CONTENTS

PART III
RESULTS

PART I

THE ISSUE

1 INTRODUCTION

The field of medicine is generally greeted with great enthusiasm —
not only by medical experts, but also by the public at large. This can
be witnessed in the immense support for medical progress in general
and the further development of individual medical research fields in
particular. It is widely hoped that these developments will lead to a
realization of idealized goals: If only medical research were to be
granted sufficient time and money, if only the secrets of the human
body were to be disclosed in their entirety, the human genome completely decoded, the most elusive physiological processes understood, then medicine would be in a position to liberate us from all the
ills of our bodily existence, if not immediately then certainly eventually. We could delay or even completely defy the aging process, for
example. We would no longer be plagued by fertility or reproduction
problems, nor pain nor other ills related to disease and dying. We
could rid ourselves of all manner of physical imperfections and even
psychological complaints. Unpleasant moods, for example, or annoy-
ing sensitivities, burdensome anxieties and obstructive irritabilities
could all become a thing of the past. The medical field would not
only be in a position to reinstate lost physical function; it could even
optimize and increase many facets of normal ability. Indeed, with the
help of medicine the human body would be controllable and con-
structible, human nature perfectible.

This book essentially sets out to examine this very idea. To encap-
sulate this notion the expression 'medical utopia' will be used
throughout this work. The excitement described is widespread,
regarding both medical progress to date and future medical
prospects. Spurred on by medical utopian fervor, the number of people who are keen to push medical progress even further is accordingly high. And yet this enthusiasm in favor of medical progress is
first and foremost a sentiment and, like all sentiments, not a product
of rational contemplation. People are capable of enthusing about the
realization of utopian notions, such as life without disease or with
the perfect body, without requiring any concrete arguments to back

them up. Enthusiasm alone is not a guarantee of ethical desirability, however. On various occasions in the past, large groups of people have become caught up in movements which have later been condemned as immoral.

So here is the problem: If we assume that this enthusiasm about the utopian prospects of modern medicine were increasingly to dispel critical reflection, then the politicians, researchers, medics and sponsors 'gripped' by this euphoria could easily become guided by it without anybody noticing, for example when establishing research priorities or distributing research funds. Without an appropriate and rational controlling mechanism, there would always be the risk of them pursuing further developments all too eagerly. And this could prove problematic. Goals of medical progress which seemed to be ideal at first sight could turn out on further scrutiny not to be at all desirable from an ethical point of view. It could also materialize that certain goals remain unattainable even after further developments in the relevant research fields, however much they were advocated at the time. In such cases the organization and funding invested in the research, not to mention possible burdens on laboratory animals and test persons, would all have been for nothing. Last but not least, there would always be the risk of various ethical problems involved in the further development and application of certain medical research areas simply being overlooked.

One of the tasks facing medical ethicists is to counteract these undesirable scenarios prospectively. For this reason it would appear beneficial to start reflecting upon the ethical desirability of developing particular medical research areas further as early as possible. Wherever feasible, critical ethical analysis should not be left until the medical technology in question is already undergoing clinical application. Otherwise ethical evaluation of the progress made in that field and its effects on humanity can only be retrospective. In this book various medical research fields will therefore be examined prospectively, in a quest to find out in advance whether developing them further would be ethically desirable or not.

To aid better understanding of the central object of this book, the first part focuses on the concept of medical utopia. It begins by defining first 'utopia' and then 'medical utopia' (Ch. 2). Next some key characteristic moments in the history of the origins of the medical utopia are presented (Ch. 3). Finally, it concludes with an explanation of the objectives and methods used in this book (Ch. 4). The second part contains a critical analysis of the ethical desirability of further developments in the following research fields: tissue engineering (Ch. 5), bioelectronic systems (Ch. 6), germ line genome modifications (Ch. 7) and interventions in the biological aging process (Ch. 8). In the last part of this book, the results of these analyses are presented and interpreted (Ch. 9). The book concludes with an appeal for ethical debate about the future course of medicine (Ch. 10).

2 BASIC CONCEPTS

2.1 Utopia and utopian thinking

At the age of 37, Thomas Morus (1478-1535) was part of a delegation chosen by King Henry VIII. In the Summer of 1515, this English contingent traveled to Flanders to meet envoys of the Duke of Burgundy, later to become Emperor Charles V, to negotiate a trade agreement. During a break in the negotiations, Morus paid a visit to the Antwerp town scribe, Petrus Aegidius. On this occasion, so Morus relates in his famous work *De optimo rei publicae statu deque nova insula utopia* (1516)[1], he met Raphael Hythlodaeus, a globetrotter and very probably a figment of his imagination. In Morus' work, Raphael describes and lauds the constitution, social order, morality, foreign policy and religion of the 'Utopians', the inhabitants of an island state called 'Utopia'. According to Raphael, the Utopians lived off the land. In their spare time they occupied their minds with humanistic studies. They practiced a religion of reason, involving modest rites and prayers. And yet they tolerated the sects which also existed there. Representatives elected by the people ruled until they died, as did their President (Morus, 1516). During the course of this dialog, Morus interrupts and criticizes Raphael, his narrator, several times. It is therefore difficult to establish with any certainty the extent to which the social form lived out in Utopia actually corresponded to Morus' own ideas of an ideal society. Morus leaves it up to the reader to decide which aspects of this *jeu d'esprit* are a true reflection of his own views and which are to be taken as intellectually stimulating humanistic wit.

Morus' neo-Latin coinage *Utopia* to describe his island state can be interpreted, on the one hand, as a combination of the Greek $o\dot{v}$ (not) and $\tau\acute{o}\pi o\varsigma$ (place, region, country). This would give 'Utopia' the meaning 'un-place', 'nowhere' or 'no-land'. On the other hand, his creation could also be formed from $\varepsilon\dot{v}$ (good) and $\tau\acute{o}\pi o\varsigma$, which

---

[1] 'On the best state constitution and on the new island of Utopia'

would result in the translation 'good place' or 'good country'. Whatever the real explanation, Morus' new word in time came to be used
to describe a particular genre of writing. To date 'utopia' has been
used in so many different contexts and for so many different works
that it is difficult to formulate a generally accepted definition of the
word (Achterhuis, 1998a). The following working definition will
therefore be used throughout this book: Firstly, the expression
'utopia' is used to describe a piece of writing which contains actual
descriptions of ideal circumstances not existing in the place and/or
at the time of the author writing the piece — for example, a state
without faults, a total domination over Nature, or a life without
death. Secondly, these circumstances of seeming perfection are themselves understood as being 'utopian'. Thus the expression is ambigu-
ous, and this ambiguity is reflected in the general use of the term.
According to this working definition, utopias existed long before
Morus thought up the name 'Utopia'. They are to be found as far
back as Antiquity (Lapouge, 1978).[2]

With regard to the localization in place and time of the ideal circumstances described in a utopia, the following development can be
observed from the time utopian thinking began in *Antiquity*: Ancient
utopian ideas were usually projected into a preceding golden age on
Earth (Ferguson, 1975). This localization pattern surfaced as early as
Ancient Greece, for example in a canonical description by Hesiod
(Works and Days), and was used well into Ancient Rome — see, for
example, Ovid (Metamorphoses, 8 A.D.). The most famous example
of a detailed Ancient utopia has to be Plato's description of an ideal
society located on 'Atlantis', an island which had sunk into the sea
long before. In the dialogs *Timaios* and *Kritias*, Plato describes in
detail a large and magnificent city situated on an island before the
"Columns of Heracles". A long time before, during "a terrible day
and a terrible night", this island had sunk into the sea. Yearning for
this golden age, Ancient man[3] gazed back in time, effectively turning
his back on the future. Plato's imagined construction was to inspire
many later utopias.

---

[2] Some authors advocate a narrower concept of utopia. They are able to recognize
utopian themes in writings from Antiquity and the Middle Ages, but in their view
"true utopia" dates back only as far as Modernity (Kumar, 1987).

[3] *Translator's note*: Throughout the text 'man' and 'mankind' are used for the German 'Mensch' and 'Menschheit' in the sense of including both sexes.

During the *Christian Middle Ages* the notion of a long-gone golden age on Earth — in the shape of Paradise — also existed, albeit accompanied by ideas about ideal circumstances projected into a transcendent future — Heaven. To a certain extent, Christian man in the Middle Ages was in a spin, fluctuating between a nostalgic look back at Paradise and hopes of eternal salvation in the next world.

The ideal circumstances to be found in *Post-Medieval* utopias were chiefly located back on Earth. On the one hand — especially at the time of the great explorers — utopias were being created along the lines of Thomas Morus' model, with the ideal situations localized in the present time and on a previously undiscovered island. On the other hand, more and more utopias were being set in the distant future, on Earth, in a non-specified location.[4] Modern man was turning his back on the past and facing the present and the future on Earth with his eyes wide open.

This is of course a simplified schema. The periods differentiated here only refer to models of utopian thinking that were dominant at that time. Yet other trains of utopian thinking continued to exist alongside them. For example, the notion of a golden age has existed into Modernity — for example Rousseau (1755) — as have ideas about an eternal afterlife in the next world. But — particularly in the industrialized world — enthusiasm for certain religious notions, as well as the hope of salvation in some kind of afterworld, have waned considerably in the course of secularization, with the result that the idea of a golden age is not nearly as prevalent now as it was in Ancient times.

Utopias are not neutral in character. To a certain extent they motivate their readers to act. After all, trying to realize the ideal conditions described in a particular utopia would seem to be an obvious step. The underlying ideals provide a certain orientation in each case. The way in which the utopian ideals in question actually motivate readers to act depends on the localization of the ideal conditions described: If — as in Antiquity — the ideal circumstances are localized in a past age, for example, then the orientation for living and acting contained within these ideals is imitation (*imitatio*). Since perfection was achieved in past ideals, a reasonable

---

[4] With regard to localization in time and space, Medieval Millennialism represented a transition between the utopian ideas of the Christian Middle Ages and those of Modernity. It proclaimed a Christendom on Earth lasting a thousand years.

course of action would be to imitate those ideals to the best of one's ability.[5]

For Christians in the Middle Ages, however, imitating the ideal circumstances of a bygone golden age was no longer an option. After all, they had considered themselves encumbered by original sin ever since Adam and Eve had been cast out of Paradise, and were thus no longer in a position to recreate the paradisical situation of long ago.[6] For Christians in the Middle Ages, life on Earth was just a transitional phase (Huizinga, 1985). However, it did determine whether at the end of time they would be experiencing never-ending Heavenly bliss or eternal damnation. Life on Earth was directed towards achieving this happiness in the next world, a true possibility provided one lived in a manner pleasing to God. There were clear guidelines and rules regarding this manner of living, to be found in the Bible (for example the Ten Commandments). Those who followed the rules could hope for a joyful afterlife in the next world. Accordingly, the God-fearing orientation for living and acting in line with Christian ideals was obedience (*obtemperatio*). From it sprang hope (*spes*) and joyful expectation (*expectatio*).

The localization of ideal circumstances in post-Medieval utopias was back in this life. Man was not only to hope for better times in the next world, but also to be stimulated to take an active part in changing his own situation. Either the utopian ideals were located in the present, but in a geographically remote place, or they were located in the future in an undetermined geographical position. These post-Medieval utopias principally functioned as critiques of the situation prevailing at the time of writing. They were supposed to motivate readers to become actively engaged in realizing the described ideal circumstances in their own present day. The orientation for living and acting during this period was reconnaissance and exploration (*exploratio*).

In the 15th and 16th centuries, the period of the great voyages of discovery, utopian works focused on the exploration of ideal societies in existence at the time of writing, yet in previously unknown, far-off locations. The idea predominated that by traveling extensively and

---

[5] The orientation towards excellence (ἀρετή) which dominated Ancient ethics was reflected in an orientation towards exemplary figures — for example people who had achieved certain forms of excellence in their lives and works.

[6] Incidentally, not even Paradise was really perfect. If it had been, original sin could not have been committed there.

exploring the globe, man could discover actual utopias. In the 17th century the emphasis shifted to geographically non-descript utopias set in the future — in other words only chronologically removed. The notion developed that man was actively capable of realizing utopian conditions of his own accord. Science rapidly advanced to become the most important means of achieving this goal. A line of thinking arose whereby a utopia could be systematically created if only science were to be suitably organized and appropriate methods applied accordingly. Scientific research, so it was believed, could enable man to change his own situation in accordance with utopian ideals. This modern idea that man has the power to create his own utopia has been triggering overwhelming enthusiasm ever since.

2.2 Modern utopias

Modern utopias began to develop in the 17th century. They contained the idea that man has the power to create his own ideal future. The following three modern utopian ideas have been cause for considerable and sustained euphoria: firstly, the idea of controlling Nature, made possible by developments in the fields of natural science and technology; secondly, the idea of shaping an ideal society on the basis of relevant theories; thirdly, the idea of controlling and constructing the human body, as well as perfecting human nature, made possible by advances in medicine.

The first of these ideas, controlling Nature using scientific and technological means, was enthusiastically received until well into the 19th century. At that time almost boundless trust was placed in promising technological achievements. The many technological achievements exhibited in London's *Crystal Palace* during the *Great Exhibition* (1851) were collectively an impressive example of the enthusiasm reigning at that time regarding man's increasing dominance over Nature. Francis Bacon's prophetic view of such dominance seemed to be receiving retrospective confirmation. Almost without exception, technological progress was celebrated everywhere as a blessing for mankind.

In the course of the 20th century, this enthusiasm about advancing dominance over Nature which had so characterized the 19th century turned into an attitude which was, if not exclusively negative, then at least exceedingly ambivalent. This development, which was to lead to the almost complete disappearance of Victorian optimism, was triggered by the First World War at the beginning of the 20th century. The battles fought brought home all too clearly the fact that new technological achievements could also be used to bring about suffering of horrific proportions. Following the shock of this war — and at the time of the Great Depression — increasingly loud voices warned of the dangers associated with progressing technology. In his *Brave New World* (1932), for example, Aldous Huxley severely criticized blind faith in progress with disenchanting pictures of an automated world. In the film *Modern Times* (1936), Charlie Chaplin depicted the depersonalizing effects of modern mass production. Following the Second World War, which revealed the terrible consequences of using nuclear arms, the utopian euphoria regarding unbridled technological progress was ultimately dampened.

Attempts to realize the second utopian idea cited above — the shaping of an ideal society — date back to the 17th century. By the end of this century numerous political modernizers and religious groups, particularly in North America, were attempting to set up small-scale utopian communities. Most of these attempts were short-lived, however. One of the best known is from the 19th century. In 1825, the British entrepreneur Robert Owen (1771-1858) founded the *New Harmony* community in Indiana. Owen's intention was to realize his own ideas regarding a comprehensive social reform. It was based on communal settlements, in which all members were to receive an equal percentage of the proceeds from their factories. Owen established the first kindergarten, the first business school and the first public library in the United States. Unfortunately, most of the approximately thousand settlers who had come to *New Harmony* at Owen's bidding were incapable of socialization, were criminal or displaced. Thus the social experiment failed, and a few years later Owen returned to Great Britain.

Enthusiasm for these small-scale utopian experiments waned somewhat following the American Civil War (1861-1865).[7] Thereafter it was new Socialist and Communist ideas which gained increasing ground. Many of the large communities founded in the 20th century on the back of these ideas lasted considerably longer than the American experiments before them. But even they have largely collapsed

---

[7] Nevertheless, new establishments of this kind have continued right up to the present day.

since. In its final throes, the Soviet Union — the Communist show-piece state — battled with immense economic problems, as well as steadily growing criticism from influential intellectuals and scientists. In the late 1980s the political leaders of the Soviet Union presented new ideas like *glasnost* (greater openness) and *perestroika* (structural reform). They declared the idea of Communist revolution to be out-dated and said that from now on the Soviet Union would step down from its traditional role as an ideological role model for World Communism. Gradually the power of Communist regimes crumbled in many Eastern European and African states. Whilst there are still Communist societies in existence — for example China, Cuba, Vietnam and North Korea — most intellectuals in modern societies today regard attempts to create a Communist remedial state as failed. In retrospect, the attempts to create utopian societies amount to a long line of failures. At the present time enthusiasm for these ideas is therefore rare. Notions about ideal social forms tend rather to be met with sobriety and reticence.

With the passing of time — and especially the 20th century — it would be true to say that enthusiasm about realizing the first two utopian ideals mentioned above dulled considerably. Both with regard to controlling Nature and to shaping an ideal society, public approval dwindled. So-called anti-utopias even sprang up as counter-reactions to that previous faith in unbridled progress. They portrayed horror scenarios of a completely industrialized world, of a society of masses dominated by totalitarianism or of the world following a nuclear war. We only have to think of George Orwell's *1984* or Aldous Huxley's already cited *Brave New World*.

A sharp contrast to that ebbing enthusiasm for the first two ideas can be seen in the widespread euphoria still meeting the utopian idea of controlling and constructing the human body, as well as of perfecting human nature. A public disappointed in its dreams of dominating Nature and creating utopian societies now appears to be directing its zeal towards this third idea. And since the medical field is believed to have the power to realize this idea — provided it may become party to the appropriate ways and means — fervor is currently aimed at a rapid advancement of this discipline.

3 MEDICAL UTOPIAN THINKING

To familiarize ourselves with medical utopian thinking, that is the modern idea of using medical means to control and construct the human body, as well as to perfect human nature, we shall start by taking a closer look at the way in which it emerged. This will not involve a detailed historical description, but a few key moments selected from the history of its origins. These key moments are followed by a number of representative examples from modern literature illustrating the way in which the medical utopia is currently presented. On the basis of these examples, a sample of the medical research fields which at present are particularly prone to inspire utopian speculations is then introduced.

3.1 Key moments in the history of the origins of medical utopian thinking

Medical utopian thinking emerged as far back as the 17th century. Prior to this, medicine, like technology and the natural sciences in general, played a very minor role in utopian thinking, if at all.[1] In the 17th century this situation changed under the influence of rapid developments in the natural sciences. As achievements mounted, particularly in the natural sciences and technology, the notions of constructibility and controllability gradually emerged: Maybe in time it would become possible for mankind to control nature in its entirety. The only fundamental requirements along the way would be that man never stopped researching, that he adopted the best possible methods and that he organized his research purposefully. Technology and the natural sciences increasingly became the subjects of utopian literature and began to instill great expectations. The dis-

---

[1] The Franciscan monk Roger Bacon (1214-1294) was a notable exception. As early as the 13th century he fantasized about ships without oarsmen, wagons that could move by themselves and machines which could fly through the air (Bacon, *circa* 1268).

coveries of Copernicus (1473-1543) and Galileo Galilei (1564-1642), for example, inspired Cyrano de Bergerac (1620-1655) to write about journeys to the moon and remote solar systems.[2]

The field of medicine also became a source of utopian ideas. The following three men in particular were to put down in words their thoughts about controlling and perfecting human nature through further medical developments: Francis Bacon (1561-1626), René Descartes (1596-1650) and the Marquis de Condorcet (1743-1794). Their works touch upon central medical utopian themes regularly to be found much later in utopian literature, albeit in different forms. Besides the prevention or curing of diseases, these themes include human longevity and the improvement of physical and mental human attributes. Since the works of Bacon, Descartes and Condorcet were to have a lasting influence on the way in which medical utopian thinking later developed, these three men can rightly be deemed its founders.

3.1.1 *Francis Bacon*

A significant point of departure for Bacon's ideas was the Christian dogma of original sin. In committing the sin, mankind forfeited not only its original innocence, but also its dominance over nature. According to Bacon, two paths could lead mankind back to the state of bliss known to Adam: on the one hand Christian faith, on the other the natural sciences. Bacon's philosophy centered on an investigation of the latter path, that of the natural sciences. He viewed them as playing a key role in the salvation of society and its members. With their help man could regain dominance over nature and many other practical advantages into the bargain. In Bacon's opinion the Ancient philosophers had not got very far in this respect, and so taking direction from them appeared to him inappropriate. He therefore believed that, if scientific know-how was to proceed in a systematic way, a whole new program had to be developed. For Bacon this implied leaving scholastic thinking behind in favor of an inductive cognitive procedure attributing key importance to observation and experiment. Bacon thus developed a methodical basis for the natural sciences of the Modernity, including the field of medicine.

---

[2] *États et empires de la lune* (1657) and *Histoire comique des états du soleil* (1662).

In *The Advancement of Learning* (1605) Bacon criticized the fact that the sciences had stood still since Antiquity. He also formulated a new way of addressing problems, as well as a prospective view of future scientific developments and their results. His work was significant for many different scientific areas; he divided science up into fields and furthermore separated it from theology. According to Bacon, science was particularly lacking in two respects. Firstly, it was not competently organized at an international level. As a result, the empirical findings of many scientists were not being adequately collated, shared and processed. Secondly, scientific objectives and methods were not sufficiently well-known (Bacon, 1605).

Bacon was to address this latter problem in his most influential work. He called it *Novum Organum* (1620) as an intended contrast to the logical and epistemological writings of Aristotle.[3] In it he explains his scientific method. He believed the essential objective of science to be dominance over nature and practical utilization of the same for the salvation of mankind. In order for science to progress purposefully towards this goal, human beings would first have to liberate themselves from prejudices of the senses and the mind.[4] Bacon also introduces the ultimate method for the pursuit of the natural sciences. He says that a good scientist is neither a metaphysicist, spinning from within himself like a spider, nor is he an empiricist, collecting knowledge like an ant. Far more he must endeavor to work through things under his own steam, like a bee. It is not enough merely to collate facts and observations without a bigger picture; instead one must proceed systematically. For science to function properly, events must be well-ordered and not confused, efficiently processed and not amateurishly. Using Bacon's method of induction, scientists should be able to proceed with caution from individual findings to more general statements pertaining to nature. These general conclusions, once thus arrived at, would then in turn lead to new experiments. In this way nature would be systematically questioned through experimentation (Bacon, 1620).

---

[3] Bacon believed the error of Aristotelian science to be the way in which definitions and theories were hastily deduced from concepts used in reference to nature and then applied back to empirical phenomena, without any way of controlling their pertinence.

[4] At this point he develops his well-known theory of the idols of the human mind (*idolae*).

Bacon chose to base his tale *New Atlantis* (1627) on these thoughts about method and organization within the sciences. In it he unfolds his design for an ideal future society, in which science would assume the position he believed it rightly deserved. Bacon's island, reminiscent of the sunken island *Atlantis* so clouded by myth, is located somewhere out in the ocean.[5] In the style of a travel account, Bacon describes how a sea-captain discovers an island on which a 'House of Solomon', named after the wise Biblical king, constitutes the central institution. This house is a well-organized scientific research center of the type necessary — according to Bacon's theory of science in *Novum Organum* — for science to progress satisfactorily.[6] In *New Atlantis* the people are occupied with the exploration of nature and the experimental production of new materials and instruments. Knowledge is multiplied systematically and interpreted by officials working on new theories. Its practical application is then overseen by different officials. Every twelve years scientists are sent to the different countries of the world. They learn the languages of these countries, observe their developments in science and technology and then return home. Here their acquired knowledge is put to good use. For the people of *New Atlantis* science is the source of happiness and wealth. This utopian research community had already mastered many technical developments which, at the time of Bacon's Europe, people could only dream about: microscopes, modern weapons, telephones, microphones, steam engines and airships, to name but a few (Bacon, 1627). Unfortunately this counterpart to Plato's tale of

[5] In writing *New Atlantis* Bacon might have been influenced by the work *La città del sole* (1623) by the Calabrian philosopher Tommaso Campanella (1568-1639), a member of the Dominican order. Campanella also chose to locate his fictitious philosophical state on an island, namely Ceylon. In his utopia the island is ruled by a High Priest elected for his outstanding scientific knowledge. He is aided by *Pon*, *Sin* and *Mor* (Power, Wisdom and Love), who in turn oversee a hierarchy of officials. It is his outstanding knowledge which prevents the High Priest from becoming tyrannical (Campanella, 1623).

[6] The description of well-organized research groups in *New Atlantis* was completely new. At the time Bacon was writing, scientists often worked in relative isolation: there were scarcely any well-organized research groups or institutes in existence. In his work Bacon anticipated the present-day scientific academies which carry out projects in the political and financial charge of the state. Just a few decades after *New Atlantis* was published, research associations began to emerge, together with their own journals in which various research findings were published. In 1660 the *Royal Society*, which had existed informally since the 1640s, was officially inaugurated by King Charles II of England. In 1671, on the other side of the Channel, the *Académie des Sciences* was founded by Colbert, a Minister under King Louis XIV of France.

Atlantis did not proceed beyond original drafts: Bacon died and it was published one year later.

One of the remarkable things about Bacon's work is that it pays considerable attention to medical research. In *New Atlantis* Bacon describes grottos, for example, in which people experiment with new methods of healing and prolonging life. The island inhabitants do the same with water from selected sources, experimenting with methods of healing and preserving health. These experiments are based on special regulation of the air in rooms built especially for this purpose. They contain large swimming pools containing various mixtures thought to heal diseases and/or improve health generally. Of particular significance are animal experiments thought ultimately to provide more knowledge about the human body and human health. To this end the island inhabitants have erected cages for all manner of animals. They study them with great precision and dissect them. They also attempt to reanimate seemingly dead animals and to manipulate by experiment the animals' growth, fertility, appearance and behavior. They attempt to cross different species, resulting in new races capable of reproducing. The results of these breeding experiments are not accidental. They are planned in advance and worked towards with purpose. The knowledge acquired about surgical interventions, medication and other curative agents as a result of various animal experiments is then applied to the human body. The island inhabitants also address dietary improvements. They make special meat, bread and drinks to render the human body more robust and enhance its performance. The cures they develop are sold by apothecaries, who stock a wide range of medicinal plants and drugs. They also have hearing aids for the deaf and hard of hearing (Bacon, 1627).

3.1.2 *René Descartes*

René Descartes' philosophy also contributed to anchoring in people's minds the concept of controlling and perfecting the human body through medicine. It is to him that we owe the image of philosophy as a tree: metaphysics as its roots, physics as its trunk and all the other sciences as its branches. These branches include medicine, mechanics and ethics. And just as the fruits of a tree are to be found on its branches and not its roots or trunk, so too, on the tree of philosophy, no real fruits are to be gained from metaphysics or physics. They have no practical application. According to Descartes, practicality is reserved exclusively for those disciplines which are last in line to be learned (Descartes, 1647). In Descartes' view, all theories within a perfect philosophy have their basis in evident metaphysical propositions, the correctness of which is beyond all doubt. In this context an important, if not the most important, philosophical aim is the good of mankind (Descartes, 1647).[7]

At the age of 41 he anonymously published his first work: *Discours de la méthode pour bien conduire sa raison et chercher la vérité dans les sciences* (1637). In this discourse Descartes describes how he was held up on the way to his military unit in the Winter of 1619/20. Sitting in a German inn near the fire, he took this opportunity to reflect upon the uncertainty of his knowledge to date and to search for new, unshakable propositions. He attempted to track these down using what he called methodological doubt. This methodological doubt permitted only things which were absolutely indubitable to be accepted as certain truths. Through this process of methodological doubt Descartes discovered that at least one truth was indubitable and therefore unshakable, namely that he himself, the doubter, existed: *"je pense, donc je suis"* ("I think, therefore I am"). With the help of this method he was therefore able to find a first absolutely certain and unshakable truth. This truth was so evident and so certain that not even the most extravagant allegation by the skeptics would be able to shake it. For this reason Descartes decided to adopt it as the first principle of his philosophy (Descartes, 1637).

On the basis of this first unshakable truth, namely that he himself existed, Descartes then introduced other truths. They included, for example, the existence of God. Here Descartes first refuted the assumption that God could be fraudulent. Since imperfection was inherent in all manners of deception, and yet God was perfect, God would not deceive mankind. Man could therefore be certain that, as long as he employed the cognitive faculties given to him by God appropriately, he would not be deceived. Human error resulted from the fact that God had given man the freedom to approve even of those things which God had failed to enable his mind to recognize clearly and distinctly. Only clarity and distinction in what is conceived could guarantee the truth of judgements then correctly made on the basis of those conceptions. Consequently, only those judge-

---

[7] From a very early stage Descartes was convinced of the primacy of applying knowledge. Cf. autobiographical references in Descartes (1637).

ments based on insight into the associations between clear and distinct conceptions could be true. Man should therefore never pass judgement on a particular matter without clear and distinct insight (Descartes, 1637).

In the fifth part of his *Discours* Descartes records that, with the help of his method and the two truths he had discovered about God and his own self, he had gone on to discover many useful and important truths about nature, the human body and the soul. His constant guides in this process were the same principles which had led him to prove the existence of God and his own self. In addition, he never allowed himself to be satisfied with conclusions of any less certainty than those permitted by geometricians. Nevertheless, circumstances had prevented him from publishing his results beforehand.[8] The sixth part of Descartes' *Discours* describes how he became convinced of the particular usefulness of his methodical principles when applying them to problems of physics. He believed them to be so productive that they should no longer be kept secret from the public. After all — unlike previous traditional and speculative philosophy — they could be made to benefit the whole of mankind. Even more than that, by applying these methodical principles, mankind could achieve dominance over nature (Descartes, 1637).

Descartes took it for granted that dominance over nature was a good thing, the idea being to invent new techniques and tricks to help make life considerably easier for mankind. The most important application for his methodical principles was the preservation of health, for in his view good health was the basis of all other goods valued by man, even their prerequisite. Since a healthy mind could only exist inside a healthy body, everything imaginable should be done to render man healthier and to enhance his performance. Descartes saw medicine as the discipline which would bring about all this. In his view, medicine may not have achieved much to date which had really benefited mankind, yet there could be no doubt that the medical knowledge in existence so far was nothing compared to the knowledge waiting to be acquired in the future. If the medical field could only gain sufficient insight into the causes of various dis-

---

[8] Descartes had actually wanted to publish his results in a work to precede his *Discours*, which was to bear the title *Le Monde*. It was nearly finished when Descartes heard of the charges against Galileo Galilei in 1633. Descartes was very moved by what happened to Galilei. He destroyed the manuscript of *Le Monde* in order to avoid a similar conflict.

eases and discover their possible antidotes, mankind could not only be liberated from physical ailments but also from diseases of the mind. Indeed, it could even become possible to eliminate the weaknesses and agonies of aging. For Descartes an elementary requirement for the development of such overwhelming medical progress was a relentless will in every coming generation to continue researching. Each generation had to pass on its knowledge to the one that followed. Descartes also regarded his own research activities as serving to empower the field of medicine in the future (Descartes, 1637).

3.1.3 *The Marquis de Condorcet*

In the 18th century, physics, chemistry and biology flourished in a manner previously undreamed of. Science and technology began their true triumphal procession. Discoveries, new theories and technical inventions in these fields were copious.[9] In the course of these developments, optimism grew regarding the notions of controlling and perfecting nature, both external and human. This environment was an ideal breeding ground for the medical utopia.

One of the encyclopedists, Marie Jean Antoine Nicolas Caritat, better known as the Marquis de Condorcet, made a very special contribution to the development of medical utopian ideas. In his optimistic work *Esquisse d'un tableau historique des progrès de l'esprit humain* (1795) he describes how the development of the human race was slowly but surely leaving the darkness and emerging into the light. The idea of progress was central to Condorcet's view of the history of mankind. In the introduction to his historical tableau of the progress of the human mind, he demonstrates why, in his opinion, the enhancement of the human race knew no intrinsic limitations. For him the human species was more or less indefinitely perfectible. The only limitation to this perfectibility was the duration of the existence of planet Earth (Condorcet, 1795).

Following this introduction, Condorcet divides history prior to his own time into nine epochs and describes how human reason gradu-

---

[9] Worthy of note here are the thermometer (Fahrenheit, 1718; Celsius, 1742), taxonomy (Linné, 1735), the kinetic theory of gases (Bernoulli, 1738), cast steel (Huntsman, 1735), the spinning machine (Wyatt, 1738), the breech-loading gun (Chaumette, 1751), the lightning conductor (Franklin, 1752), nitrogen (Rutherford, 1772), the theory of combustion (Lavoisier, 1780), the hot-air balloon (Montgolfier, 1783) and animal electricity (Galvani, 1790).

ally developed with the natural progress of civilization. There were some crucial junctures at which human progress ascended to a higher level: families joining to form tribes; man dropping hunting in favor of cattle farming and agriculture; the alphabet being invented, etc. In the tenth book of his discourse, Condorcet addresses the future. Based on collated historical findings, here he attempts to take some threads further. He sees three important lines of development: the realization of equality between individual countries; the realization of equality between different peoples; the perfection of human nature (Condorcet, 1795).

In his sketch on the future progress of the human mind, Condorcet describes how, to a certain extent, future realization of equality between all human beings had to be a prerequisite for achieving the highest level of human perfection. In his opinion, sustained peace, a flourishing economy and scientific achievement were all built on the elimination of obvious inequalities between human beings. At the same time, sustained peace, a flourishing economy and scientific achievement would encourage further perfection in human individuals. At the end of his description of the progress of the human mind, Condorcet describes the benefits which mankind could hope to reap from progress in the medical field. Together with improvements in hygiene (both for the body and for human dwellings) and in diet, plus some lifestyle changes (for example avoidance of extreme exertion), medical progress would ensure that in the future human beings lived healthier and longer. Medical progress would even ultimately lead to the disappearance of all infectious diseases, as well as diseases caused by unhealthy climate, poor diet or excessive labor. All remaining diseases would also disappear as soon as mankind had tracked down their causes and eliminated them (Condorcet, 1795).

The further perfectibility of the human species would be almost unlimited. In time mankind would even conquer the aging process. Human beings would probably not become immortal, but the average human lifespan could be expected to extend indefinitely. In the future mankind would be able to live without disease and without physical defects, and would be able to enhance its performance beyond all limitations. In his exposition Condorcet included observations on animal experiments, on the heredity of characteristics from parents to children, and on the ways upbringing influenced human beings. He was convinced that different strengths acquired by an individual — for example increased resilience or sharpened senses, as well as greater intelligence or even improved morality — would be passed on to that person's children. Accordingly, the perfecting of human beings could continue forever (Condorcet, 1795).

3.2 Current medical utopian ideas

From the moment the first medical utopian ideas emerged, the discipline of medicine was assigned enormous potential. At that time it was *de facto* capable of very little. The general lack of medical skills and expertise meant that it was reduced to the alleviation of symptoms and moral support for patients. Initial enthusiasm surrounding the potential of medicine was therefore based chiefly on all manner of theoretical considerations and extrapolations. Today this has fundamentally changed. Many of the medical utopian ideas popular today are based not on theoretical mind games, but on a rapid succession of real scientific achievements.

The course taken by medicine began to speed up in the 19th century. The possibilities of anesthesis and asepsis facilitated the development of new invasive surgical techniques. In the 20th century, the discovery of penicillin and other antibiotics, as well as the introduction of sulfonamide, meant first successes in the cure of bacterial diseases. Medical diagnostics was rendered more sophisticated by the development of ultrasound, computer tomography (CT), magnetic resonance imaging (MRI), scintigraphic techniques, endoscopy, as well as immunological and molecular biological methods. Many new medical disciplines emerged, for example brain, heart and lung surgery, transplantation medicine, psychiatry, works medicine, preventive and social medicine, sports medicine, reproduction technologies, neonatology, geriatrics and human genetics. This increase in the range of medical activity has resulted in the intensive way in which in the Western world the medical profession tends to stick close to human beings — from the moment they are born until the moment they die. These new options have of course also meant a very real increase in the capabilities of modern medicine. And this evident capacity of the discipline, with its ever-growing and seemingly unlimited possibilities, has in turn had a stimulating effect on public euphoria. In view of how much medicine has achieved within such a short space of time already, present-day man loves to speculate about its ongoing potential.

The key issues addressed by the founders of the medical utopia —
namely the prevention and cure of diseases, extension of the lifespan
and the improvement of physical and mental human attributes —
have hardly changed today. What has drastically changed, however,
is the circumstance that they are now linked to real and substantial
medical developments and progress. Enthusiasm is no longer
reserved exclusively for theoretical considerations and hypothetical
mind games; present euphoria is chiefly directed at real-life medical
research fields.

Something which has not altered over the years is the fact that it is
not only medics, i.e. specialists from within the discipline, who are
euphoric about current medical developments: Authors who do not
deal with medicine in any professional capacity are choosing to write
enthusiastically about the potential of modern-day medicine; and the
public at large is also increasingly enthusiastic about the spectacular
medical progress being made.

In order to give an impression of how the key medical utopian
issues are being linked in the literature to actual medical progress
and developments, there follows a small selection of relevant works.
This selection does not presume to present the whole range of current
medical utopian thinking in its entirety. And yet it does intend to
give a good impression of the variety and range of ways in which
the key issues of medical utopian thought are currently being
addressed. The first two works selected were written by medics, the
last three by authors from outside the medical field.

3.2.1 *Life without Disease. The Pursuit of Medical Utopia*

In his book *Life without Disease. The Pursuit of Medical Utopia* (1998),
medic William Schwartz takes a retrospective and prospective look at
medical developments between 1950 and 2050. He assumes that various
long-standing utopian notions will soon become reality as a
result of explosive growth in genetic expertise. In view of the developments
to be expected, he urges that the social and economic consequences
be considered now (Schwartz, 1998).

According to Schwartz, between the years 1950 and 2000 considerable
successes were marked up in diagnostics and the elimination
of defects caused by disease. And yet the old utopian notions have
only been partially realized as a result of this progress. In Schwartz'
view this is mainly due to the fact that during those fifty years medicine
concentrated less on fighting the causes of disease and more

on eliminating its consequences and symptoms. Between the years 2000 and 2050, however, mankind will succeed in combating the causes of health-related defects. This will happen as a result of developments in molecular medicine, combining the expertise of genetics and molecular biology. By developing this medical field further, mankind will be in an increasingly better position to comprehend the genetic causes of health-related defects. On the basis of this extended knowledge, new methods of disease prevention will then be developed for people with certain genetic predispositions (Schwartz, 1998).

Schwartz goes on to predict that man will steadily increase his knowledge about the processes which lead from an unfavorable genetic structure to pronounced disease. This will present him with an ever-growing number of ways in which to utilize molecular interventions in order to disrupt these destructive processes. Schwartz believes the therapeutic potential of molecular medicine to be so enormous that a child born in 2050 may well have a life expectancy of 130 years. It will also probably not have to suffer from any of the most prominent chronic diseases of our time. For the first time ever, and in the not-too-distant future, the discipline of modern medicine will provide a scientific basis for the realization of old utopian notions (Schwartz, 1998).

3.2.2 Reversing Human Aging

The possibility of increasing human life expectancy far beyond the normal range assumes an important role in many medical utopian ideals. In connection with this ideal, growing biomolecular expertise is a particular source of optimism. In his book *Reversing Human Aging* (1996), medic Michael Fossel attributes a key role in the aging process to so-called 'telomeres'. Telomeres are the two end-pieces of a chromosome. Every one of the 46 chromosomes has a telomere at each end. A telomere comprises the last few thousand DNA bases, plus the corresponding proteins. Telomeres become shorter with every cell division. On average, telomeres lose approximately fifty base pairs every time a cell divides (Fossel, 1996).

According to Fossel, once the telomeres of a cell have reached a critically short length, cell division slows down until it ultimately stops altogether. A cell like this then sends out 'help signals' to its neighboring cells, setting various reactions in motion. For example, the signals trigger the release of inflammatory mediators or the production of inflammatory cells like macrophages. These do not only damage the cell in question, however, but also its immediate vicinity. According to Fossel, aging cells also cease being able to react adequately to the signals of other cells. As a result, they are no longer able to fulfill 'their obligations' to their neighboring cells. The damage is thus able to spread and what begins as localized episodes builds up to produce cumulative consequences. At first the functions of individual tissue parts and organs are affected, then ultimately the whole body. In Fossel's opinion, age-related changes first affect cells which are dividing. Secondary damage may also be caused to cells in their vicinity which have ceased to divide. The shortening of the telomeres is thus the cause of cellular aging, which in turn is the most important factor for the aging of the overall body, as well as many of its diseases. Thus telomeres are the main cause of the aging process and its related diseases (Fossel, 1996).

In his exposition about the aging process, Fossel attempts to provide a foundation for a correct understanding of treatments which will intervene in the biological aging process and which, in his opinion, will soon be available. In his eyes, telomerase will play a major role. Telomerase is an enzyme which can lengthen telomeres. Fossel believes that, with the help of this enzyme, an aged cell can be made young again. Lengthening its telomeres would enable the cell to resume its normal cellular cycle. Since telomerase is not present in most cells naturally, it would need to be properly introduced. Venous administration is not a particularly promising option: The enzymes usually found in human blood would quickly break down the telomerase. The half-life of telomerase in human blood is therefore very short. However, Fossel states, various alternatives to venous administration would be conceivable: Firstly, a telomerase equivalent, a synthetic telomerase which is more robust and stable than the natural form, could be used; secondly, special genes could be manufactured which would be in a position to generate telomerase inside human body cells, maybe thus enabling the cells to lengthen their own lifespan; thirdly, and this is the option most favored by Fossel, the genes already present inside human cells could be stimulated to produce telomerase. This would involve developing a telomerase inductor, a substance which could be injected into a cell to stimulate the production of telomerase there. Thus therapies to delay the aging process of human cells could be developed, with the ultimate aim of prolonging human life (Fossel, 1996).

In addition, Fossel writes, telomeric manipulation could mean treatment for diseases such as cancer, premature senility and vascular conditions. A cancer therapy could be developed using telomerase inhibitors, for example. Substances would be injected into a cancerous cell to inhibit the production of telomerase. The aim of this treatment would be to prevent the excretion of telomerase and to destroy cancerous cells. According to Fossel, the manipulation of telomeres could also be useful in conjunction with breeding organs. Using this enzyme, a tissue part could continue growing outside the body forever, provided the cell culture is nourished accordingly. In this way all tissue types could be produced in the required quantities (Fossel, 1996).

Fossel's belief is that first attempts at telomerase therapy in human beings will begin by 2005. By 2010 this form of therapy will probably be generally available. In the two decades thereafter it will become possible to combat many severe diseases, as well as to intervene in the aging process at will. In the long term mankind will thus largely be liberated from disease and pain, as well as live longer. In Fossel's opinion mankind can expect a life which is vital and almost never-ending (Fossel, 1996).

3.2.3 *Remaking Eden. Cloning and beyond in a Brave New World*

As has already been mentioned, progress in modern medicine has also inspired authors not directly involved in the medical field to write optimistically about the constructibility and controllability of human nature in the future. One such author is Lee Silver, Professor of Molecular Biology in Princeton. In his work *Remaking Eden. Cloning and Beyond in a Brave New World* (1997) he expounds upon the utopian notion that future parents will be able to decide the genetic make-up of their own children. 'Reprogenetics', a label coined by Silver, will provide them with this option. This future discipline is based, on the one hand, upon the enormous progress being made by reproduction medicine. Silver is led to assume that within the foreseeable future every couple or individual — regardless of sex or age — will be able to have its own biological children. On the other hand, it is also based on rapidly growing expertise in the field of genetics. Silver assumes that utilization of state-of-the-art computer technology in genetics will in time facilitate the development of DNA chips which will be able to scan an entire human genome both quickly and inexpensively. Large-scale population studies, identifying connections between genetic patterns and phenotypical characteristics, would then be possible. According to Silver, man will thus in time comprehend the links between physical or mental characteristics and gene profiles (Silver, 1997).

The aim of reprogenetics, so Silver states, is to guarantee or hinder the heredity of particular genes. Reprogenetics is concerned with the issue of which genes will be passed on to an individual child. An example Silver gives of a gene with desirable heredity is the AIDS resistance gene. Currently only about one per cent of the population possesses this totally harmless gene rendering its carrier resistant to HIV. Using gene technology a child could be equipped with the AIDS resistance gene. Silver believes that in the longer term reprogenetics will enable prospective parents to add entirely new genes to the genomes of their children. This will give them a better chance of having healthy, prolonged and successful lives. In addition, Silver believes that prospective parents will in time be able to decide which of their own genes they would like to pass onto their children and which not. All manner of individuals and couples will use the new techniques in order to achieve aims which could not be achieved otherwise. In Silver's opinion, reprogenetics will mean increased reproductive freedom. It will give people the chance to have happy, healthy and successful children (Silver, 1997).

Silver outlines the way in which these options could develop as follows: For security reasons — to avoid side-effects — only genes occurring naturally in human beings would be used at first. These could be genes to increase life expectancy, to diminish aggression, to promote musical prowess, to facilitate the learning of a foreign language or to minimize shyness. As experience grows in the medium term, characteristics and abilities currently not possessed by any living human being will be made available. Silver assumes that no techniques will be used before they have been proven safe and viable in animal experiments. The benefits of these new technologies will far outweigh any risks they might involve (Silver, 1997).

Silver does believe reprogenetics to be problematic in one sense, namely that less wealthy families and social groups who cannot afford such applications will be in danger of becoming seriously disadvantaged. He follows this with the comment, however, that wealthy parents in America today can already buy better healthcare and education for their children than their less wealthy peers. The children of wealthy parents already grow up in an environment

which in many ways encourages later success. So why should repro-
genetic applications be forbidden when they merely have the same
effect (Silver, 1997)?

Overall, the use of reprogenetics could have considerable consequences for society and humanity: If there were to be no legal restrictions imposed on reprogenetics — which Silver incidentally assumes
— free markets within society would in time lead to a gulf between
two classes of people, the genetically enhanced and the natural
human beings. According to Silver, the direction which this development would then take would be determined by the market, i.e. the
interests of the individuals and couples themselves, as well as those
of their children. Silver expects that mankind will change his own
biological foundations to such an extent that in the future two human
species will exist side by side, the *GenRich* and the *Naturals* (Silver,
1997).

3.2.4 *Visions. How Science will Revolutionize the 21st Century*

In his foretelling scientific report *Visions. How Science will revolutionize the 21st Century* (1997), Michio Kaku, Professor of Theoretical
Physics in New York, claims that with the end of the 20th century science has reached the end of an era. According to Kaku, the 20th century was particularly characterized by progress in three significant
scientific areas, namely quantum physics, genetics and computer science. As a result of this progress, the basic laws governing matter,
life and calculation have now been explained. Mankind has split the
atom, examined the molecules of life and created the electronic computer. In Kaku's opinion the era of great discoveries is now drawing
to a close, and the era of controlling and utilizing the technologies
stemming from these discoveries is beginning. Kaku believes that in
this dawning new era man could reap the benefits of two thousand
years of scientific work. Man's status regarding nature is ceasing to
be that of a mere observer and is in transition to becoming that of a
controller. For this new era Kaku has various exciting prognoses,
based among other things on insights gained from exchanges with
over 150 prominent researchers over many years. His predictions
mainly apply to the next 100 years (Kaku, 1997).

First Kaku addresses the developments which rapidly advancing
computer technology will bring about, for example in the field of
bionics. By about the year 2020 it may be possible to link silicon
microprocessors embedded in artificial eyes, legs or arms directly to

the nervous system. In this way paralyzed parts of the body could be reactivated and enormous relief brought to the disabled, for example. Kaku also describes the fusion between man and machine which he believes to be just around the corner. In time it will become possible to transfer the consciousness of a human being to a robot with no loss of consciousness for the human being as a result. Using a special, complex procedure, a surgeon could very gradually, and without consciousness being lost, replace the human brain by a mass of electronic neurons. The technology required to perform such a procedure might be located far into the future, and yet, Kaku emphasizes, human beings should already begin deciding whether in the future they would like to become 'cyborgs' (human machines) or not (Kaku, 1997).

Kaku also addresses radical changes in the field of molecular biology. He concentrates on the future consequences of these outstanding biomolecular developments. Kaku predicts that in the third decade of the 21st century we will be able to compile individual DNA codes. These individual DNA data will then, according to Kaku, revolutionize the way in which diseases are dealt with. With the help of new therapies, for example gene therapy or the utilization of 'intelligent molecules', man will be able to cure many previously incurable diseases, for example various forms of cancer. In addition, by 2020 the genomes of viruses and bacteria will be mapped in their entirety. Using this information, new insights will be gained into the manifold mechanisms by which various pathogens gain entry to the human body. Man will also comprehend how they reproduce within the human organism and cause damage (Kaku, 1997).

Following these explosive steps forward, Kaku believes that other developments will be much slower in coming. It will probably not be that easy or even possible to automate the analysis of gene functions and interactions and thus have the task performed by a computer. And yet sooner or later mankind will understand the varied interactions between genes. On this basis man will then be in a position to treat polygenic diseases more effectively. Kaku also predicts great progress in the manufacture of transgenic organisms. However, modification of hundreds or even thousands of genes within one organism will probably not be achieved before the end of the 21st century. We will probably have to wait several centuries for the arrival of the *homo superior*. After all, thousands of genes will have to be manipulated for its creation (Kaku, 1997).

Concerning the treatment of problems linked to aging, Kaku favors hormone therapy. In his opinion, in the next decades it could well be used to halt various age-related decaying processes. Hormone therapy could also provide protection from certain diseases. But the human lifespan will remain unchanged. From 2020 research will begin to discover aging genes. The knowledge thus gained will then serve to delay or even repair the molecular damage brought on by aging. Should aging genes actually be found to exist, and should their manipulation enable human beings to live longer, then new organs will probably be required to replace old ones which have worn out. After all, it is far from certain whether manipulation of aging genes would render the body young again. The field of tissue engineering is already investigating techniques by which new tissue parts and organs can be generated in the laboratory. According to Kaku, by the end of the second decade of the 21st century we will be able to buy many different organs and tissue types: skin, bones, vascular valves, ears, noses and maybe even livers and kidneys. By 2050 we will be able to manufacture more complex organs and whole body parts, such as hands, hearts and internal organs. After that we will probably be in a position to replace any organ within the body (Kaku, 1997).

3.2.5 *The Age of Spiritual Machines*

In his work *The Age of Spiritual Machines* (1999), the computer scientist Ray Kurzweil presents his view that in the 21st century the dividing line between human and artificial intelligence will become increasingly blurred. Before the 21st century draws to a close, mankind in the form familiar to us today will no longer be the most intelligent creature on earth. Even now a large and ever-increasing number of tasks previously reserved for human intelligence is being performed by computers. The superiority of computer intelligence regarding speed, reliability and memory capacity will become increasingly obvious in the course of the second decade of the 21st century. Computers will be integrated in human clothing, acting as health monitors, diagnosing diseases and providing recommendations for treatment. The vital processes encoded in the human genome will become transparent — especially the information-processing mechanisms which are presumed to underlie degenerative diseases and aging. Average life expectancy will rise to over 100 years (Kurzweil, 1999).

Kurzweil goes on to predict that by the end of the third decade of the 21st century most limitations associated with disability will have been eliminated, made possible by specialized neuroimplantation technologies, among other things. Blind people, for example, will have at their disposal highly intelligent navigational aids. The physically disabled will have intelligent orthopedic prostheses to stimulate their nervous systems. And deaf people will have access to display devices capable of transcribing the spoken word. In addition, many people will use devices to increase their sensory abilities. A multitude of neural implants will be available to enhance memory and logical thinking. Knowledge will continually grow about the ways in which the genetic code controls the processing of information. In the course of this development mankind will better his understanding of age-related afflictions and dysfunctions and thus be able to treat them more effectively. Kurzweil believes that as a result the average life expectancy will increase to about 120 years. Additional ways of prolonging life will focus on the mass use of bionic organs. So-called 'nanorobots' will be used to construct these organs, which will be capable of repairing themselves if damaged (Kurzweil, 1999).

Kurzweil defines nanorobots as miniscule, intelligent machines which can copy themselves, solve all manner of problems and alter their surroundings. Once integrated in the human blood circulation system, he believes they could complement the natural immune system, as well as eliminate a large number of harmful factors — e.g. fatty deposits in the arteries, cancerous cells and pathogens. With the help of this technology man will be in a position to reconstruct every organ and system within his body. With the aid of more flexible and durable materials human beings will also be able to redesign every single cell making up the various organs and tissue types. Stronger and more efficient organs will thus be constructed (Kurzweil, 1999).

Due to the exponential increase in computing capacity, Kurzweil predicts a rapid improvement in the resolution and speed of scan technologies. In the 21st century it will become possible to map the various regions of the human brain, synapse for synapse. With the aid of these technologies, man will then be able to create artificial neuronal networks which will function very similarly to certain aspects of human intelligence. Furthermore it is conceivable that man will succeed in mapping the position, connections and contents of every neuronal component within the brain — cells, axons, dendrites, presynaptic vesicles, etc. Once all the individual parts of the brain have thus been recorded, its organization can then be reconstructed on a 'neuronal' computer (Kurzweil, 1999).

Kurzweil believes it possible that in the second half of the 21st century more and more aspects of human intelligence will be transferred to machines: Each specialized region of the brain will be scanned and its function analyzed and interpreted. Following this, corresponding artificial counterparts will be produced and can then be added to according to the most diverse of wishes. Intelligent systems will thus be developed which, besides having the advantages of speedier data processing and greater data processing capacity, will also be qualitatively improved compared to human, organically organized intelligence. By the year 2100 an individual human being will be able to transfer his entire consciousness to a computer file and add new capabilities to it at will. Software-resident intelligences will then emerge, claiming to be persons. The number of such artificial intelligences will rapidly exceed the number of human beings still using the organic method of data processing. The people still using their organic brains to think will, however, also increasingly use neuroimplants in order to enhance their sensory and cognitive abilities. The software-resident intelligences will be able to manifest themselves in bodies as they please. The bodies will either be produced using nanotechnology or will exist at different levels of virtual reality. In the context of these software-resident intelligences, the traditional concept of life expectancy will lose all meaning (Kurzweil, 1999).

3.3 Main research fields

These five selected works from the literature give a good idea of the spectrum of current medical research fields addressed by present medical utopian thinking. A closer look permits a division of these various medical research fields into three categories. The first category contains research fields already in clinical application and includes all those developments already tested on human beings or implemented as treatments. The second category is that of research fields at the preclinical stage and includes those developments already being tested on cells or tissue *in vitro*, or on animals, but which have yet to undergo clinical trials. Accordingly, the findings from these research fields have yet to play a role in current clinical practice. The third category contains research fields which, to date, remain purely theoretical, including every speculative, hypothetical edifice of ideas. These research fields are concerned with theoretically conceivable medical developments for which not even the initial stages of practical work have been attempted.

These three categories of medical development can now be assigned to actual medical research fields which have a particular tendency to encourage utopian ideas. The research fields 'tissue engineering' and 'bioelectronics', both already in clinical application, would fall into the first category, for example. Tissue engineering is concerned with the breeding of cells and tissue parts as biological replacements parts, to be used in the reconstruction, maintenance or enhancement of various bodily functions. Some of these biohybrid products are already in practical use. In the area of bioelectronics, various bioelectronic systems — i.e. systems linking electronics with living tissue — have been developed. Here too, research findings have already led to clinical applications, for example cochlea implants in the ear.

The second category, that of developments at the preclinical stage, includes research fields like 'reproductive cloning', 'germ line genome modification' and 'interventions in the biological aging process'. In the area of reproductive cloning — referring to the production of a genetically identical organism (called clone) from another organism using asexual reproduction — techniques are currently being developed which would mean an expansion of the possibilities offered by reproduction medicine to date. The field of germ line genome modification researches possible ways of bringing about genetic changes within an organism which can then be passed on to its descendents. It is hoped, for example, that such interventions will facilitate the prevention of certain diseases across several generations.[10] Last but not least, the area concerned with interventions in the biological aging process is researching possible ways of influencing the human aging process. The techniques currently under investigation could in time lead to prolonged human life expectancy. In all three of these medical research fields cited, developed techniques have already been used on animals, with varying degrees of success.

---

[10] First germ line genome modifications have already been performed in clinical practice as part of infertility treatment. Ooplasm has been transplanted from a donor egg cell to the egg cell of a prospective recipient mother (see 7.1.4).

The third category, that of developments which so far remain purely theoretical, includes research into the possible development of nano-sized, computer-controlled machines to perform all manner of medical interventions (1 nanometer [nm] = 1/1000 micrometer). This is by far the most speculative of the research fields addressed here. It is concerned with theoretically viable medical applications as a result of nanotechnology research findings. Complete concepts for medical nanomachines capable of acting independently and equipped with molecular motors, as well as special vehicles and sensors to locate desired targets, are already available on paper. According to the 'nanomedics', such machines would facilitate extremely precise interventions at cellular and molecular levels, thus considerably expanding the current range of medical possibilities. In practice, however, nanometric constructions of this kind have yet to be realized.[11]

In Part II of this book we will take a closer look at four research fields often refered to in the utopian literature: 'tissue engineering', 'bioelectronics', 'germ line genome modification' and 'interventions in the biological aging process'. They will serve as a basis for analyzing whether ethical arguments can be found to support the noted euphoric advocacy of the further development of these fields.

A passing comment: Dystopian mistrust of medicine

This description of the various reactions provoked by the rapid progress of medicine would be one-sided if it concentrated exclusively on utopian euphoric reactions and completely omitted those of dystopian mistrust. Amongst other things, dystopian fears can be seen as a dialectic reaction to the — in their perception exaggerated — euphoria of the advocates of modern medicine. The utopian euphoria tends to drown out such negativity; in certain societies, however — like Germany, for example — dystopian mistrust of medicine represents a significant countermovement.

---

[11] However, the vast majority of current nanomedical research projects is focusing on a great variety of simpler nanostructures. Freitas (2005) distinguishes 96 subcategories of current nanomedical research projects. Among them are projects as diverse as studies of raw nanomaterials, nanostructured materials, control of surfaces, nanopores, DNA manipulation and sequencing, tools and diagnostics, intracellular devices, BioMEMS, nanotherapeutics and nanorobotics. A large number of scientists — affiliated both to universities and to private companies — are currently occupied with a great number of different potential medical nanotechnology applications. This research is already affecting a variety of different medical sub disciplines.

Within the various dystopian expressions of distrust one or more of the following three motives can often be heard: The first motive is a fear that modern medical research, especially in the field of genetics, could lead to a reanimation of eugenic ideas. The eugenics paradigm was developed as early as the 1860s by the Englishmen W. Greg, A. R. Wallace and F. Galton and spread rapidly to various Western countries. Supporters of this new discipline, the so-called 'eugenicists', shifted values in the following radical way: They made the individual recede behind the 'genus' and then abstracted from the former to the species or 'race'. What mattered was the qualitative composition of the genetic material of the population. They also increasingly propagated the political maxim that the interests of the present generation were to bow to those of future generations. Eugenic population policy was more or less becoming official. It provided biologistic solutions to the 'social question' of how best to deal with the social problems of the time caused by industrialization (Weingart et al. 1988).

In the United States, in the first half of the 20th century, eugenic population policy led in some states to the passing of sterilization legislation. The eugenics which emerged in Germany towards the end of the 19th century, also known as 'racial hygiene', particularly in the works of Alfred Ploetz and Wilhelm Schallmayer, was from the start more radical in its objectives than Anglo-Saxon eugenics (Weingart et al. 1988). From the outset the notion of killing human beings for 'selection' reasons played a role as a means of implementing policy. And yet this notion was on no account at the center of the racial hygiene program. In the first decades of the 20th century other methods of implementing eugenics were widely discussed, too. They included restricting preventive and welfare measures in classes of the population deemed 'genetically inferior', in order to increase their death rate. Other points were the creation of marriage prohibitions for the 'genetically inferior', banning them to special homes and/or sterilizing them in order to prevent them from reproducing. One of the most radical implementations of German eugenics has to be the 'euthanasia practices' of the National Socialists (Nazis) (Schmuhl, 1986). With this in mind, some authors view certain aspects of modern genetic research as an impermissible breaking of a taboo. They see it as having parallels to the eugenics movement of that time and fear a renewed development of certain eugenic ideas (Höhn, 2000; Poliwoda, 1992).

A second motive for dystopian mistrust is irresponsible medical research. This negative picture of medicine partly arose due to the increasing information gained over the second half of the 20th century about the role of certain physicians in the National Socialist era. The horrific details of National Socialist medical experiments on human beings (Proctor, 1988) shocked the world. Numerous immoral medical experiments gradually came to light, not only in Germany, but also, for example, in the United States and Great Britain. To a certain extent medicine lost its innocence in the 20th century.[12] These terrible events in the area of medical research made everyone aware that the conducting of extremely immoral medical experiments can be a reality.

The third motive for dystopian mistrust is the increasing commercialization of medical research. More and more commercial enterprises now conduct their own research. In addition, firms regularly choose to finance research projects which are in their own interests. One of the chief motivating forces behind this commitment is the hope of profit. Some writers in the literature now fear that the temptation of potential profit could become so dominant that in the future more and more research projects will be conducted without any thought for ethical norms. They worry that commercial enterprises involved in research projects could conveniently ignore certain ethical norms in order to reap the desired gains as speedily as possible (Andrews & Nelkin, 2001; Kimbrell, 1993). Despite all this, dystopian mistrust towards modern medicine is not the concern of this book. For this reason the individual aspects of this phenomenon will not be examined any further.

---

[12] Modern research ethics emerged as a reaction to these shocking experiences. It began with the so-called 'Nuremberg Codex', which was passed in 1947 in the light of the horrors of the medicine of the Nazi regime as an internationally valid ethical basis for all medical research. Following various debates and changes to this Codex, generally accepted norms now exist for experiments on human beings (for example informed consent or proportionality between risks and benefits).

4 CRITIQUE OF THE MEDICAL UTOPIA

4.1 Study objectives

It is understandable that euphoria is incited by the utopian idea of being able to use medical means to control and construct the human body, as well as to perfect human nature, so encouraged as it is by medical progress. The number of people who applaud medical progress and who are keen to see further developments in this area is therefore correspondingly high. And yet, as described earlier, it would seem dangerous to allow this feeling of exultation to become so predominant that ethical reflections on medical developments are completely overshadowed. Fired by utopian enthusiasm, politicians, researchers, sponsors, clinicians and patients could, in the course of such a development, blindly follow where this feeling leads, a feeling which has wholly or partially circumvented critical reflection. This could in turn mean the fevered encouragement of additional medical developments which, from an ethical point of view, might be wholly undesirable.

This book is an attempt to counteract precisely this danger. It investigates the ethical desirability of further developments in those medical research fields which are currently particularly prone to encouraging medical utopian notions. The result will be a critique of medical utopian thought from an ethical point of view. The analysis will concentrate on four key medical research fields, all encouraging utopian notions and all introduced earlier, namely tissue engineering, bioelectronics, germ line genome modifications and interventions in the biological aging process. These research fields have all been specifically selected as representatives of the enormous spectrum of medical research fields which are currently inciting utopian euphoria.

4.2 Method of analysis

For further developments in a particular medical research field to be deemed ethically desirable, the following three conditions must be fulfilled:

Condition 1: The objectives underlying further development of the medical research field must be worth striving for from an ethical point of view.

Condition 2: Further development of the research field must actually contribute to a realization of these objectives.

Condition 3: Any ethical problems concomitant with the further development and application of the medical research field must be justifiable or surmountable.

Each one of these three conditions is equally as important as the other two. After all, each one individually represents a prerequisite for the desirability of developing a research field further. If, for example, the first condition were not fulfilled, further development of the research field would mean an envisaging of objectives which are not ethically desirable. If, however, the second condition were not fulfilled, the objectives would be desirable, but further development of the research field would not enable them to be realized. And if the third condition were not fulfilled, the objectives would be both desirable and realizable following further developments in the research field, but the concomitant ethical problems would be unacceptable. The further development of a research field cannot be deemed ethically desirable in any of these three situations. This means that if a particular research field fails to fulfill just one of these conditions, its further development is automatically ethically undesirable.

An investigation into the desirability of further developments in a particular medical research field therefore has to be carried out by checking whether these three conditions are all fulfilled. This will be done in Part II of the study, addressing each one of the four above-mentioned medical research fields individually: tissue engineering, bioelectronics, germ line genome modifications and interventions in the biological aging process. The following three questions need to be posed in order to determine whether the three conditions are fulfilled:

Question 1: Are the objectives behind a further development of the research field really desirable from an ethical point of view?

Question 2: Will further development of the research field really contribute to a realization of those objectives?

Question 3: What ethical problems are to be expected from a further development of the research field, and are they justifiable or surmountable?

Each of the four individual research field analyses begins with a description of its two most significant objectives. These are chiefly taken from the literature, which varies in volume depending on the research field in question. The three questions are then answered in order, individually for each of the two objectives behind the research field in question.

Analysis of the first question is elementary in light of the fact that an objective may only appear desirable *prima facie*. The first question will be answered using three answer categories, depending on the result of the analysis: 1) The objective is really desirable; 2) it is not clearly desirable; 3) it is not desirable. Each of these possible answers has a corresponding consequence as far as the first condition is concerned: 1) The condition is fulfilled; 2) its fulfillment is problematic; 3) it is not fulfilled.

Overview of possible results upon answering the first question:

Objective:	Fulfillment of the first condition:
really desirable	Yes
not clearly desirable	Problematic
not desirable	No

In order to analyze the second question — whether further development of the medical research field will really contribute to a realization of the objective in question — the medical literature is consulted, which varies in volume depending on the field. Depending on the result of this analysis, here too the answer may fall into one of three categories: 1) It is certain or at least very probable that further development of the research field will contribute to a realization of the objective in question;[1] 2) the contribution is uncertain; 3) further development of the research field will not or at least very improbably contribute to a realization of the objective in question. Again, each of these possible answers has a corresponding consequence as far as the second condition is concerned: 1) The condition is fulfilled; 2) its fulfillment is problematic; 3) it is not fulfilled.

---

[1] It does not seem reasonable solely to demand *certain* contribution to the realization of an objective, as further scientific development cannot be predicted down to the last detail, on principle (Popper, 1982).

Overview of possible results upon answering the second question:

Contribution to realization of the objective in question:	Fulfillment of the second condition:
certain or very probable	Yes
uncertain	Problematic
non-existent or very improbable	No

In order to analyze the last of the three questions — whether ethical problems concomitant with further development of the research field in question are justifiable or surmountable — a differentiation is made between three different problem categories. These categories essentially serve to elucidate the problems described in the medical ethical literature. They do not claim to be absolute, nor to provide clearly defined divisions for all ethical problems. The first problem category contains ethical problems obstructing a particular medical technology from being developed responsibly and/or implemented appropriately (Have, 1995; Have et al. 1998). A typical problem in this category might be the major risks involved in applying a technology from a particular research field. The prerequisites for responsible development and appropriate use when dealing with a technology play a key role in the assessment of this category of problems. These ethical prerequisites will therefore be scrutinized in the course of the analysis. Various ethical evaluation criteria already exist, including risk assessment, informed consent in clinical research and proportionality between the risks and benefits of applying a particular technology.

The second problem category contains ethical problems which are intrinsically linked to the technology itself and which are thus independent of whether or not the requirements for its responsible development and appropriate use are complied with during the development and/or application of that technology. They refer to infringements of ethical dictates or prohibitions which necessarily accompany the development and/or application of the technology in question. One example of this problem category would be the regularly debated problem of destroying and/or instrumentalizing embryos in the context of the research field of therapeutic cloning and its further development (see 5.4.2). The problems falling into this category will be referred to in this study as 'problems intrinsically linked to the technology'.

The third and last problem category defined here in the context of further developing a particular medical research field concerns the negative effects it could potentially entail in the long term. The problems included in this category are, firstly, so far in the future that they cannot be included in the potential consequences of a new medical technology usually taken into account in the context of responsible development and appropriate use (e.g. in the assessment of risks). Secondly, they are not — in contrast to the problems in the second category — intrinsically connected to the further development and application of a particular technology. Examples of this third problem category would be changing human attitudes to the human body potentially resulting from further technical and scientific successes in the research field of tissue engineering (see 5.4.3).

For an analysis of the last of the three questions — whether and to what extent the ethical problems concomitant with further development of a medical research field are surmountable and/or justifiable — the medical ethical literature is consulted, which varies in volume depending on the research field in question. An extensive debate is published for the research field of germ line genome modifications. In contrast, ethical discussion about interventions in the biological aging process is much less developed. And regarding bioelectronics and tissue engineering, ethical reflection is only just beginning.

The following three answer categories will be used for the results of this analysis: 1) The ethical problems concomitant with further development appear to be surmountable and/or justifiable; 2) it appears uncertain whether they can be surmounted and/or justified; 3) the problems do not appear to be surmountable and/or justifiable. The first answer will only be permitted where a) a new technology can be developed responsibly and/or used appropriately; b) there are no or solely negligible problems intrinsic to that technology; c) potentially negative effects in the long term are either non-existent, very improbable or avoidable. The second answer is appropriate where there is serious doubt as to whether the conditions a), b) and/or c) can be fulfilled. The third answer is given where at least one of the three conditions can definitely not be fulfilled. Each of these possible answers has a corresponding consequence as far as the third condition is concerned: 1) The condition is fulfilled; 2) its fulfillment is problematic; 3) it is not fulfilled.

Overview of possible results upon answering the third question:

Ethical problems are surmountable and/or justifiable:	Fulfillment of the third condition:
Possible	yes
Uncertain	problematic
not possible	no

If the overall analysis should reveal that *one or more* of the three conditions cited *cannot be fulfilled* with regard to an individual objective behind a medical research field, then this book will evaluate the further development of this research field as *ethically undesirable* as far as this objective is concerned. If the result of this analysis is such that whilst, with regard to an individual objective behind a medical research field, none of the three conditions is unfulfillable, the fulfillment of *one or more* of the three conditions is *problematic*, then this book will evaluate the *desirability* of developing this research field further, as far as that objective is concerned, as *questionable*. The further development of a research field will only be evaluated as *ethically desirable* or, to put it more precisely, *principally* ethically desirable with regard to a particular objective if *all three* conditions are *fulfilled* for this objective.

With regard to a particular objective behind a medical research field:	Ethical desirability
One or more conditions are not fulfilled	no
Fulfillment of one or more conditions problematic	questionable
All three conditions fulfilled	*principally* yes

The qualification 'principally' is crucial. After all, the principal desirability of developing a medical research field further with regard to an individual objective means: (1) The objective is worth striving for; (2) further development of the medical research field will definitely or very probably contribute to the realization of this objective; (3) further development *can* proceed in a manner ethically justifiable. This does not necessarily mean that it will actually *happen*. Thus if the further development of a medical research field regarding an individual objective is deemed 'principally ethically desirable', this does not automatically mean that all conceivable ways of developing this field further are ethically desirable.

4.3 Ethical viewpoint

This book is subtitled "Ethical Observations". Since a whole spectrum of different ethical viewpoints exists, this section will detail the specific viewpoint underlying this study. It is customary for the presentation of a particular ethical stance to be preceded by the ethical principles supporting this view. Such principles are fundamental. They are characterized by the fact that they are not in turn based on other, more general principles from which they can be deduced. Ethical principles are the ultimate yardstick for ethical evaluation. They can be used as arguments to support subordinate ethical norms or singular moral judgements. Examples include the Stoic principle "Live life in accordance with nature" and the utilitarian principle "Always endeavor to act in such a way as to bring the greatest happiness to the greatest number of people". Ethical principles often play a key role in ethical analyses.

However, calling upon ethical principles entails the following two elementary difficulties: Firstly, finding rational justification for their validity is still problematic. Within the discipline of ethics, opinions therefore differ regarding whether, and if so how, the validity of certain ethical principles can be justified. Secondly, the suitability of using ethical principles as a crutch when reaching actual moral decisions is rightly doubted (see 4.3.1). In the light of these difficulties, this book does not seek orientation in any particular set of principles. Instead, the ethical viewpoint underlying this investigation is conditioned by the following three assumptions:

Firstly, it is assumed that, in order to reach a verdict about the moral aspects of a particular circumstance (for example how good, bad, permissible, condemnable or valuable it is), it is vital that the overall situation in which the circumstance arose is taken into consideration. The moral aspects of a particular circumstance, e.g. a particular action, are not identical in every situation. They depend on other circumstances influencing the situation and are thus conditioned by the context of the situation in question. Thus ethical principles are of little — if any — use when forming moral judgements. After all, such principles presuppose identical moral aspects for a certain circumstance at all times, which is just not true within our multifaceted moral reality. This first assumption appears in the literature as *particularism*.

Secondly, this book assumes that moral judgements are neither exclusively, nor primarily, irrational displays of emotion or incitements to act. Instead, they make statements about reality. A reality is presupposed which, in addition to its physical, chemical, biological and psychological aspects, also has its moral aspects. Moral statements refer to moral aspects. They may correspond to the moral aspects existing in reality or they may not. Accordingly, the statements are therefore true or not true. In ethical terms, this second assumption can be described as a combination of *cognitivism* (moral statements are either true or not true) and moral realism (a reality containing moral aspects exists).

Thirdly, this book is based on the assumption that it is fundamentally impossible to say for sure whether a moral statement is actually true or not. The criteria required in order to establish its truth beyond any doubt do not exist. In contrast, it is possible to establish the untruth of moral statements in certain cases, for example when they are logically inconsistent. For this reason, moral statements are to be viewed as well-founded hypotheses. This last assumption could be termed a mild form of *skepticism*.

An adequate substantiation of the three abovementioned assumptions would exceed the framework of this critical analysis of medical utopian thought. However, they are explained below in more detail.

4.3.1 *Particularism*

Particularism states that when moral judgements are being made about particular circumstances, the focus must always be on the situation in which these circumstances occurred. The moral aspect of a particular circumstance is always partially determined by the context of the situation in which it took place. As a result, the same individual circumstance — for example, a particular act — is fundamentally capable of having different moral aspects, depending on the situation.

This can be illustrated by the act of lying, the conscious telling of an untruth. Imagine the following three different situations: In the first situation a person has just sworn to a court to tell the truth, the whole truth and nothing but the truth; in the second situation a person is being tortured in the hope that information about friends of his will be gained; and in the third situation a test person is taking part in a psychological experiment, the research protocol of which demands of test persons that they lie about certain things. Particularists believe that although the same act is performed in each of these three situations, namely lying, different moral aspects are attributed to it in each case. The reason for this is that the moral aspect of the act of lying is fundamentally inseparable from the circumstances of the individual situation. It is elementarily linked to the context of the situation in question. If the situation changes, the moral aspect of lying changes with it.

The moral aspects of circumstances therefore possess a variability which is situation-bound. In ascertaining the moral aspects of a particular circumstance, it is therefore only consistent to adopt not an atomistic, but rather a holistic approach, i.e. one which takes into account the overall context of the situation in question. Bearing this in mind, particularists are reluctant to deploy ethical principles, believing them to represent generalized judgements about the moral aspects of certain circumstances in an infinite number of situations.[2] Generalizing statements presuppose that a particular circumstance always has the same moral aspects in the most varied of contexts. Particularists cannot accept this. In their view, moral reality is so complex that it is fundamentally impossible to comprehend it adequately using ethical principles. The moral aspects of a particular circumstance, or so they believe, are partly influenced by the associated circumstances of the situation in question and are thus subject to a context-dependent variability that cannot be adequately grasped by principles (Dancy, 1993; McNaughton, 1988).

In the branch of particularism underlying this book, ethical principles are not divested of their usefulness altogether, however. Provided they are used cautiously, they can prove helpful in the course of moral considerations as *rules of thumb*. They can function as heuristic aids, helping moral decision-makers to distinguish between the essential and the non-essential, or drawing attention to certain morally relevant points.[3] Of course, such heuristic rules of thumb do not always point in the most suitable direction.

---

[2] In the so-called *universalistic* theories — for example, Kant's ethics or utilitarianism — certain ethical principles are granted absolute validity. If, for example, lying is evaluated in a universalistic theory as being morally reprehensible due to a corresponding principle, then every act involving lying is automatically deemed immoral. By contrast, in *generalistic* theories ethical principles are only valid *prima facie* (cf. Ross, 1930). Theories like this invite moral conflict. It is conceivable, for example, that in a concrete situation two different ethical principles may both be valid *prima facie*, demanding two different mutually exclusive manners of proceeding. In such cases the situation must be analyzed in order to determine which of the two principles is more momentous in the case in hand.

[3] Whenever principles are referred to in this book, they are always to be taken as heuristic rules of thumb.

In the forming of a moral judgement about a particular circumstance in a certain situation, a key role is played by so-called *moral
competence*. It is chiefly characterized by the following elements:
1) moral sensitivity 2) moral argumentation and 3) moral experience.
Moral sensitivity is the ability to pick up on the moral aspects of different circumstances in a situation and to weigh them up against
each other before pronouncing a moral verdict. Following on from
the moral aspects gleaned from that particular situation, first moral
considerations can then take place. *Moral argumentation* plays a crucial role here, as well as in any later justifications of moral decisions
made. The long-term product of repeated moral decision-making in
a wide variety of situations on the basis of sensitivity and argumentation is *moral experience*. This is knowledge about the various moral
aspects of particular circumstances occurring in different contexts.
This knowledge is hard to systematize without losing any of its complexity and richness. However, on the basis of moral experience it is
possible to draw up certain heuristic rules of thumb for the moral
evaluation of individual circumstances in a certain type of situation.
Moral experience plays a part in every moral verdict reached.

4.3.2 *Cognitivism and moral realism*

This book has its foundations in moral realism. According to this
school of thought, reality does not only have its physical, chemical,
biological and psychological aspects, but also its moral aspects
(McNaughton, 1988). In addition to the views of moral realism, this
book also embraces those of cognitivism. Cognitivists believe that
moral judgements are not exclusively or primarily irrational displays
of emotion or incitements to act. Far more, they make claims about
reality. Moral statements are therefore propositions. In contrast to displays of emotion or incitements to act, propositions can either be true
or untrue; which one depends on whether the proposition is in agreement with reality or not (cf. Kutschera, 1982).[4] In this study moral

---

[4] For a better understanding of cognitivism, it is worth taking a look at its counterpart, non-cognitivism. According to the non-cognitivists, moral statements on no
account serve to make claims about reality. They may appear as propositions in their
external grammatical form — e.g. "Killing is immoral" — and yet the function of
moral statements is not to claim that particular facts exist. Their character is far more
that of wishes or commands. In the first sense, as wishes, they — just like expressions of consent, aversion or bitterment — are therefore only an expression of the
subjective *attitude* of the person making the statement. As such, they can really be

realism and cognitivism are combined. It is assumed that moral statements are true whenever they describe moral aspects — existing in reality alongside physical, chemical, biological and psychological aspects — precisely as they are. If the description does not fit, they are untrue.

4.3.3 *Skepticism*

It is by no means always possible when reaching a normative verdict in a situation requiring a decision to pay sufficient attention to all the morally relevant aspects of that specific situation, or to include them in one's considerations leading up to a moral decision. To illustrate this, we only have to look at the reaching of normative decisions in clinical or political practice. In both of these areas moral decisions regularly have to be made in highly complex situations with little time to spare and on the basis of limited factual knowledge. Perfect conditions for the forming of moral judgements in such situations — such as peace and quiet, time for reflection and sufficient documentation — rarely exist. In addition, those who have to pronounce moral judgements are not always party to sufficient moral sensitivity, moral argumentational skills or moral experience. It may thus be assumed that human normative decision-making necessarily involves an element of fallibility.

In practice, absolute certainty as to whether a pronounced moral statement is true cannot be fundamentally claimed to exist. The reason for this is that there are no criteria for establishing the indubitable truth of pronounced moral judgements. In this book, moral statements are therefore consistently regarded as hypotheses. This is true both for specific moral statements and *a fortiori* — due to the assumed variability of the moral aspects of a circumstance depending on its context — for general moral verdicts.[5]

---

said to have a primarily *expressive* component. Commands, on the other hand, — just like directives, instructions and recommendations — really serve the person making the statement only as a means of inciting to a particular action. As such, they primarily have an *evocative* component. According to the non-cognitivists, a descriptive component (a claim that certain facts exist) is either totally lacking in moral statements, or it is completely overshadowed by the expressive and/or evocative dimension (cf. Ayer, 1936; Hare, 1952; Stevenson, 1944).

[5] This view of moral statements as having the character of hypotheses is not intended to imply pragmatism. An elementary difference between the latter and the view presented here can be found in the truth theory. In pragmatism a statement has to prove itself in practical terms and over time before it can be deemed true; in the

By contrast, in some cases it may be possible to establish the indubitable untruth of a moral statement. Take, for example, moral statements which can be proven to contain a moral inconsistency. Or verdicts based on facts which later turn out to be quite different from those assumed at the time the verdict was reached: these too can clearly be disqualified as untrue. If, for example, historiography should unearth new facts in conjunction with a particular historical event, giving that event a different moral relevance, then all moral judgments previously accepted for this event must be declared untrue and altered accordingly.

4.3.4 *The reaching of moral decisions on the basis of moral uncertainty*

As detailed above, the three cited assumptions do not permit moral certainty. They do not allow life to be led or actions to be perpetrated according to indubitably true moral insights. And yet this lack of absolute moral certainty should not lead one to the fatalistic assumption that it is fundamentally impossible to raise the quality of human moral decision-making.

The following two factors refute this assumption. Firstly, the moral competence playing a key role in the forming of a moral judgement about a particular circumstance in a specific situation is not an unchanging constant. Its three most important elements — moral sensitivity, moral argumentation and moral experience — can be improved upon. *Moral sensitivity* can be trained by observing the way in which already morally sensitive persons arrive at moral verdicts in specific situations. Close cooperation with a morally sensitive senior consultant could mean, for example, a considerable improvement in the moral sensitivity of an intern just starting out in clinical practice. *Moral argumentation* is an intellectual skill, and as such one which can be improved with suitable instruction and sufficient practice. Finally, *moral experience* can be gained by immersing oneself consciously in all areas of life, taking in its entire breadth and depth and ultimately looking critically at all the different moral issues which surface in the process.

The second factor which refutes the fatalistic assumption that it is fundamentally impossible to raise the quality of human moral decision-making refers to the way in which the process of normative

ethical viewpoint defended in this book, however, truth is only determined by whether or not a statement accurately describes moral reality.

decision-making is organized in specific situations. If, namely, this process is organized in an appropriate manner, the quality of moral considerations and decisions can be raised quite considerably. Proper organization, in the author's opinion, begins with a clear description of the ethical problem at hand. It then continues with a listing of all the relevant facts. This not only does justice to the complexity of the situation; it also enables the moral aspects of all its different circumstances to be ascertained. On the basis of these facts a discursive process should then take place, in which the moral considerations resulting from the moral aspects of the various circumstances are weighed against each other. The moral statements emerging from this discourse, which might take place within a single person or within a group, must be allowed to compete freely with each other. On the one hand this increases the chance of untrue moral statements being identified as such and excluded; on the other hand, by excluding untrue judgements, those moral verdicts which remain in the running conversely have an increasingly large chance of actually being true — in that the rational means at the disposal of the ethical debate are not actually able to disqualify them as being untrue. At the end of this process an argumentatively justifiable decision can then be reached.[6]

Against the background of the ethical viewpoint outlined here, the moral verdicts reached in this book should be viewed as well-founded hypotheses on which to base a more extensive debate. The situations addressed by this book, such as state-of-the-art research in selected scientific fields, are complex. Various future scenarios are analyzed, none of which can, at the present time, be free of vagueness or uncertainty. It therefore seems only consistent to view the moral statements made in this study as hypotheses, a point worthy of repeated emphasis. Instead of claiming them to be true, the author wishes them to be an inducement to prolonged critical debate.

---

[6] The last few decades have witnessed the development of methods for multidisciplinary ethical case analysis in clinical practice, enabling the quality of moral decision-making in clinical practice to be raised. In problematic cases these methods envisage a joint compilation of all the relevant facts by all the persons involved in treating the patient in question, from their different disciplinary points of view. This is then followed by an argumentative debate on the morally relevant aspects of the problematic situation, in which these aspects are weighed up freely against each other (Steinkamp & Gordijn, 2005).

4.4 Relevance of this book

If medical ethics wishes to be of any relevance in conjunction with the rapid progress being made by medical research and technology, the following two points seem to be elementary: 1) Medical ethics should analyze the various moral aspects of medical research and technology prospectively; 2) In addition to the issue of responsible development and appropriate use, it should also address and analyze the issue of the desirability of medical technologies (Have, 1995; Have et al. 1998). These two points are described in more detail below.

1) As far as the first of these two points is concerned, medical ethicists are faced with the following dilemma. If they reflect upon the potential future practical applications of certain medical research fields before they are actually available, their considerations are in danger of being dismissed as pure speculation and thus not reputable. They are viewed as something akin to science fiction. If, on the other hand, medical ethicists wait until medical research findings are available and the technology has already found its way into clinical practice, then they may be accused of closing the stable door after the horse has bolted. Their ethical considerations — which might have been helpful prior to the introduction of the technology in question — are too late. Afterwards they have next to no practical relevance.

Thus if medical ethics really is to be of practical relevance, the indications are that it must dispose of any fears that its considerations could be dismissed as non-respectable speculation. This is significant because only a continued prospective painting of existing medical research trends, followed by an ethical analysis of their various aspects and consequences, can facilitate advance regulative intervention — in accordance with the ethical insights gained. In addition, anticipative ethical analysis appears to be indicated when — as is the case with the medical research fields analyzed in this book — the application of certain research findings could have far-reaching consequences for mankind. Especially in cases such as these, ethical reflection should not wait until research is completed and findings are clearly revealed in clinical applications. This book supports medical ethics being of practical relevance. It analyzes *prospectively* various ethical aspects surrounding the development and application of technologies from four different medical research fields. It thus facil-

itates advance regulative intervention in these four research fields —
should the ethical insights gained indicate it.

2) Ten Have (1995) categorically demanded that medical ethics
address and analyze not only issues of responsible development and
appropriate use, but also issues of the desirability of medical technologies. According to Ten Have, issues of responsible development
and appropriate use center around the problem of how exactly the
responsible development of a specific new medical technology and
its careful and attentive application should unfold. Adopting this
approach, both further development of the technology itself and its
subsequent clinical application are just assumed as facts, without any
critical reflection. In Ten Have's eyes, evaluating a new medical technology in this manner means observing it 'from the inside'.

Issues of desirability, on the other hand, center around the problem
of whether, and if so to what extent, the technology in question is
worth striving for and thus permissible at all. Adopting this
approach means looking at a technology 'from the outside', so to
speak. It means questioning whether it is appropriate for a technology to exist at all. It means, for example, investigating the precise
moral concepts underlying an emerging technology and subjecting
them to a critical ethical examination. According to Ten Have, neither the development nor the application of a medical technology
takes place within a moral vacuum. Certain values — such as
'increased knowledge' or 'reduced suffering' — are always being
attributed to them and influencing them. By questioning the fundamental desirability of a technology, these values are no longer just
blindly assumed, but are critically examined. In addition, this process
involves an investigation into whether further development and subsequent application of a particular technology could possibly
encroach upon any other values. Issues of desirability therefore call
into question whether it is appropriate for a new medical technology
to exist at all (Have, 1995; Have et al. 1998).

If medical ethics wishes to be of practical relevance, it should
therefore, in addition to the matter of 'prospectivity', take to heart
this second point. It should address not only issues of responsible
development and appropriate use, but also and especially issues of
desirability. Ten Have gives the reason for this as follows: In limiting
an analysis purely to responsible development and appropriate
application, medical ethicists observe new medical technologies
exclusively 'from the inside'. This does not grant them the distance

necessary for critical reflection. This kind of medical ethical observation could be fatal, however, leading to medical ethics being instrumentalized to suit the purposes of those interested in furthering the
development of a new technology, and being misused by them as a
means of asserting their own interests, namely a smooth realization
of the objectives behind the medical technology in question. It would
also mean elementary medical ethical issues being swept under the
carpet, such as the fundamental question of whether a particular new
medical technology is desirable at all, or a critical investigation of the
objectives subliminally pursued by this new technology. These questions only come to light if a technology is observed 'from the outside', with the necessary critical distance (Have et al. 1998).

Regrettably, or so we learn from Ten Have, present-day medical
ethics is still strongly oriented towards analysis of issues related
purely to the responsible development and appropriate application
of medical technologies. Its traditional approach to date has been
geared chiefly to the manner in which particular research projects
and their practical applications must be organized in order to proceed with a maximum of care and attention. In so doing, medical
ethics is unfortunately occupied very one-sidedly with presenting
and assessing various problems related to the responsible further
development and appropriate clinical application of new medical
technologies, as well as with the search for possible solutions to these
problems. To date the issue of desirability has been addressed far too
infrequently (Have, 1995; Have et al. 1998).

This book endeavors to contribute to reducing this shortcoming.
Its aim is to pursue — in addition to the point of 'prospectivity' crucial to practical relevance — this second abovementioned point in
particular. Its central theme is that of desirability, examining the issue
of whether and to what extent the further development of certain
new medical technologies and their clinical applications can really be
deemed *desirable* from an ethical point of view. Developing and
applying a new medical technology in a responsible manner does
represent a necessary condition for the desirability of taking that
technology further, it has to be said. And yet, as has been said
already, other crucial conditions exist, too: The objectives behind this
technology really have to be ethically desirable; further development
of the technology must make a real contribution to realizing these
objectives; and finally, not only the problems relating to the responsible further development and appropriate application of the tech-

nology must be justifiable, but also the problems intrinsically linked to the technology itself and the problems connected to the consequences of the technology in the long term. An ethical approach directed one-sidedly at the analysis and solution of problems relating only to responsible development and appropriate use would therefore obstruct a more fundamental and complete analysis. It is even true to say that solving these problems is of no real interest until all the other conditions providing an argumentative foundation for the ethical desirability of a technology have been fulfilled.

In summary, this book is firstly a plea for a wider use of prospective analyses in the ethical evaluation of new medical research projects and technologies. Secondly, it is a plea for medical ethics to find its direction in a questioning of the fundamental desirability of developing certain medical research fields further. Instead of living more or less in symbiosis with the field of medicine — as it has often appeared to do in the past — medical ethics should become a clearly distinct entity. After all, critical reflection always requires a certain amount of distance to its object. Instead of remaining put in its current position of an auxiliary science to medicine, medical ethics should become the 'thorn in its side'. It is the only way it will be able to contribute to its improvement in a manner both substantial and long-term.

PART II

ANALYSIS

5 TISSUE ENGINEERING

5.1 Research field

5.1.1 *Tissue Engineering*

The idea of creating human tissue and organs or even a complete human being dates back as far as the Biblical tale of the creation of Eve. This story — emerging around the time of Solomon (972-932 B.C.) — reports that God created another person from Adam's rib, 'a woman brought unto the man' (Gen 2, 21f). A more modern example of creating human beings dates back to 1818: Mary Shelley's novel *Frankenstein*. Here the creative experiment is performed not by God, but by man himself. It was not until a few decades ago that the idea of creating human tissue and organs emancipated itself from the realm of imaginative fiction and became a dynamic scientific field. This new medical discipline is now known as 'Tissue Engineering'. A first definition of this research field was put forward at a symposium held in California in 1988:

> "Tissue Engineering" is the application of principles and methods of engineering and life sciences toward fundamental understanding of structure-function relationships in normal and pathological mammalian tissues and the development of biological substitutes to restore, maintain, or improve tissue functions. (Skalak et al. 1988, xx).

Later definitions of this new discipline have especially stressed the last aspect — the development of biological substitutes to restore, maintain or improve tissue functions — and the interdisciplinarity of the field. Tissue engineering is primarily viewed as an interdisciplinary science which is occupied with the breeding of biological substitutes to restore, maintain or improve tissue and organ functions (cf. Desai, 2000; Nerem, 2000; Patel et al. 2002). One example of research in this field is the laboratory production of complex, three-dimensional tissue — literally a copy of human tissue design and function. The complexity of this process requires the deployment of different scientific disciplines. Major roles are played by principles and methods from both the life and engineering sciences (thus the name tissue *engineering*).

A significant motivating force behind the development of this new discipline has been the increasingly urgent problem of organ shortage (Fuchs et al. 2001; Risbud, 2001; Stock & Vacanti, 2001).[1] Developments within this research field took a noticeable leap forward in the 1990s (cf. Vacanti & Vacanti, 2001). By 2001 approximately 3,300 scientists and assistants were working with tissue engineering and its potential applications in more than seventy companies worldwide. In the year 2000 these companies invested approximately US$ 600 million in the development of new products (Griffith & Naughton, 2002). The overall capital invested since 1990 has exceeded US$ 3.5 billion (Lysaght & Reyes, 2001).

5.1.2 *Techniques*

A fundamental distinction can be made between three different tissue engineering procedures currently under development (Griffith & Naughton, 2002; cf. Fuchs et al. 2001; Langer & Vacanti, 1993; Risbud, 2001). These three procedures are *in situ* tissue regeneration, the implantation of cells or small cell clusters, and the utilization of 'biohybrid' or 'bioartificial' systems.

In the first of these techniques, *in situ* tissue regeneration, individual molecules, for example growth factors, are introduced directly into the defective body tissue. The molecules then stimulate the body's endogenous cells to regenerate the desired tissue (Mooney & Mikos, 1999). A variation on this procedure involves implanting a scaffold, bathed in the relevant growth factors, within the damaged tissue. Here too, the growth factors stimulate regeneration of the tissue locally. The scaffold thus used to create new tissue degenerates at a later date (Babensee et al. 2000; Griffith & Naughton, 2002).

Various methods exist for implementing the second technique, the implantation of cells or small cell clusters. One of these methods is the injection method. It involves injecting into the patient

---

[1] In 1989 there were 19,095 patients on the waiting list for an organ transplantation in the U.S.; eleven years later this figure had risen to 71,366 patients (Nasseri et al. 2001).

individual cells of desired tissue. The cells thus introduced to the recipient tissue then become active and organized within that location. New tissue begins growing within the body, using surrounding vessels and connective tissue for stabilization and as a mold for its reorganization (Pollok & Vacanti, 1996). Another method for implanting cells or small cell clusters is the *in vitro* seeding of cell aggregates on biodegradable scaffolds, which are then implanted in the defective tissue (Griffith & Naughton, 2002). A further development has been the so-called 'closed system method' (Risbud, 2001; Vacanti & Langer, 1999). The name derives from a treatment using cells encapsulated inside a membrane which is non-permeable for certain sizes of molecule. The membrane surrounding the cells permits diffusion of nutritional and waste products, but cannot be permeated by larger molecules such as antibodies or immunological cells (Fuchs et al. 2001; Lysaght & Aebischer, 1999). An advantageous side-effect of this method is that the semipermeable membrane also shuts out potentially carcinogenic cells (Pollok & Vacanti, 1996). Parallel to the implantation of individual encapsulated systems, tissue engineers are also working on extracorporeal systems. One example of this approach would be efforts to develop extracorporeal liver replacement systems, aimed at finding a solution to the problem of acute liver failure (Lysaght & Aebischer, 1999). Acute liver failure is a disease with a high mortality rate. To date the only treatment is emergency liver transplantation. An extracorporeal liver replacement system could help bridge the time to transplantation. Following the transplantation of a donor liver, it could then continue to provide support during patient regeneration (Heath, 2000).

The third technique, utilization of 'biohybrid' or 'bioartificial' systems, is aimed at the manufacture of long-lasting, living replacement organs and tissue. In this technique individual cells are isolated from the desired tissue and then applied to special, three-dimensional, artificial constructions. The idea is then to control their reproduction and encourage them to become living tissue. Suitable materials for the scaffolds on which the cells are to multiply would be biodegradable, natural materials, such as collagen, or synthetic polymers. 'Biohybrid' or 'bioartificial' systems are implanted in the recipient organism and there assimilated. As this last technique is probably the most spectacular of the three, it is worth taking a closer look at how it works.

5.1.3 *Biohybrid tissue and organs*

The manufacture, still in its early days, of spatially defined tissue, organoid structures or even complete organs[2] for implantation can be described as follows (cf. Minuth, 2002; Patel, 2002). Firstly a sufficient number of cells from the envisaged tissue-specific cell type must be harvested. This is done by performing a biopsy on the appropriate part of the donor organism. Autologous or allogenous human somatic cells are currently used as starter cells (Vacanti & Langer, 1999).[3] Allogenous cells are used in cases where the tissue recipient does not have enough healthy cells for a cell sample (Curtis & Riehle, 2001; Heath, 2000).[4] The sample is then cleaned of unwanted cells and fed with growth or serum medium in conventional culture dishes to encourage proliferation (Strehl et al. 2002). During this process the differentiated cells can rapidly de-differentiate. Compared to their natural environment, their artificial environment is less complex. As a result, differentiated cells can lose many of their special functions *in vitro* which they have *in vivo* (Luyten et al. 2001; Risbud, 2001; Stark et al. 2000b; Vacanti & Vacanti, 2000). In order to avoid or reverse this situation, an environment has to be created which imitates the natural environment of the culture cells. A template is needed to guide new growth from the isolated cells (Stark et al. 2000a & b). The latter do not possess an intrinsic tissue structure. A histoconductive support is thus introduced to the artificially enlarged cell cluster to guide the regeneration of tissue structure in the cell cluster. The support consists of an extracellular scaffold with a corresponding — two or three-dimensional — structure (Curtis & Riehle, 2002; Nimesh et al. 2002). The materials used for this scaffold have to be highly porous, biocompatible and biodegradable (Fuchs et al. 2001; Hutmacher et al. 2001). Materials can be either natural or synthetic (Yang et al. 2001 & 2002). The cell culture is pipetted onto

---

[2] Various problems are still hindering the *de novo* breeding of complete organs in purely artificial surroundings (see 5.3.1).

[3] Latest developments in the harvesting and breeding of pluripotent stem cells (see 5.1.5) have given rise to the idea that this type of cell could possibly be used in the future to manufacture complex tissue groups or entire organs. To date, next to no experience is available in connection with use of this cell type to manufacture tissue or organs, however. Current experience is limited to fully differentiated cells and adult stem cells (Bianco & Robey, 2001).

[4] In the future it may also be possible to correct certain genetic defects using genetic engineering methods (Shay & Wright, 2000b).

this scaffold, which creates and maintains enough space for the cells to form. Its structure both controls development and permits diffusion of nutrients. Seeding the cells within the scaffold plays an important role in their formation according to tissue type (Hutmacher et al. 2000).

The necessity of controlling the way in which the tissue and its special characteristics develop is the pivotal feature of this method. Implants are expected to have the typical characteristics they would have in their natural environment. For control purposes the scaffold containing the cells is often not kept conventionally in a cell culture. Instead — to make things easier — it is placed in a tissue holder and this in turn is placed in a perfusion culture chamber or bioreactor (Strehl et al. 2002).[5] The latter ensures that cell cultures are permanently perfused with fresh culture medium. The aim behind these perfusion chambers is to simulate whichever environment is typical for the tissue in question (Fuchs et al. 2001; Griffith & Naughton, 2002). By permanently renewing the culture medium the supply of nutrients can be controlled, and by adding soluble differentiation factors and hormones to the culture medium differentiation can be controlled more extensively (Fuchs et al. 2001; Strehl et al. 2002). In time a biohybrid formation appears. Growth can be observed in microscope chambers. The seeded isolated starter cells move into the three-dimensional scaffold and begin to grow in accordance with the space available. Gradually the cells fill up the scaffold. No longer needed, the biodegradable scaffold then dissolves. Ideally it melts away gradually, optimizing tissue shape (Curtis & Riehle, 2001).

5.1.4 *Current tissue engineering applications*

Current research in the field of tissue engineering is concerned with nearly all tissue and organ types. The development of relatively primitive replacement tissue, such as skin or cartilage tissue, is already pretty far advanced. Clinical trials with biohybrid replacement skin tissue are already taking place. This kind of replacement tissue is used in the treatment of complex wounds, skin cancer or severe burns (Fuchs et al. 2001; Johnson, 2000). The first product manufactured using tissue engineering, *Transcyte* (Naughton, 1999),

---

[5] Cited attempts with bioreactors are still predominantly experimental (Curtis & Riehle, 2001).

was a skin replacement product from the firm *Advanced Tissue Sciences*. In 1997 it was authorized for sale by the *Food and Drug Administration* (FDA). Other examples of skin replacement products include *Dermagraft* (Naughton, 1999), also from *Advanced Tissue Sciences*, or *Apligraft* (Parenteau, 1999), manufactured by the firm *Organogenesis*. Clinical trials are also going ahead with replacement cartilage tissue possessing the desired elastic structure. One example of this kind of replacement tissue would be the product *Cartical* from the *Genzyme Corporation*. Replacement cartilage tissue is used in reconstructive surgery, for example in the treatment of injured or altered joint surfaces (Kim & Han, 2000). In the future replacement cartilage tissue could also be used in ENT surgery (ears, nose and throat).

In addition to research projects to develop replacement skin and cartilage tissue, numerous other tissue engineering projects are researching the manufacture of replacement tissue products. They include projects to develop biohybrid replacement tissue for bones (Braddock et al. 2001; Musgrave et al. 2002), for the liver (Nasseri et al. 2001; Terada et al. 2000), for the pancreas (Risbud, 2001), for the intestine (Terada et al. 2000), for heart valves (Mann & West, 2001), for the heart (Akins, 2002; Zimmermann et al. 2002), for blood vessels (Mann & West, 2001; Nerem & Seliktar, 2001), for the esophagus (Fuchs et al. 2001), for the trachea (Fuchs et al. 2001), for the cornea (Risbud, 2001), for the retina (Layer et al 2002), for the breasts (Shenaq & Yuksel, 2002) and for the bladder (Gustafson & Kratz, 2001; Yokoyama, 2001).

Bearing this wide range of research activities in mind, it is reasonable to expect that the rapidly developing field of tissue engineering may in time influence all manner of medical disciplines in clinical practice. Examples include dentistry (Hillmann & Geurtsen, 2001), urology (Yokoyama, 2001), orthopedics (Musgrave et al. 2002), pediatric surgery (Grikscheit & Vacanti, 2002) and plastic surgery (Friedman, 2001).

5.1.5 *Stem cell technology*

Thanks to recent developments in the field of harvesting and breeding embryonic stem cells, speculation abounds as to whether in the future this specific kind of cell might not be used to manufacture certain cell types, tissue groups or even entire organs (Chapekar, 2000; Cibelli et al. 2001 & 2002; Fuchs et al. 2001; Griffith & Naughton, 2002; Heath, 2000; Lanza et al. 1999b; Odorico et al. 2001; Pedersen,

1999; Suh, 2000). Compared to embryonic stem cells, the fully differentiated cells used to date have one big disadvantage: their limited ability to multiply (Curtis & Riehle, 2001; Fuchs et al. 2001; Luyten et al. 2001; Noishiki, 2001). Embryonic stem cells, by contrast, seem to be able to go on dividing indefinitely (Wiestler & Brüstle, 2002). They also seem to be capable of differentiating into many different cell types (Rohwedel, 2001). Scientists even believe that the self-renewal and differentiation skills of embryonic stem cells could render them a more or less limitless donor pool for transplantation medicine (Denker, 1999; Heath, 2000). If it became possible to control their differentiation, it would in time also become possible to manufacture in the laboratory, for example, nerve cells for Parkinson's sufferers, heart cells for heart attack victims, insulin-forming cells for diabetics and blood-forming cells for leukemia sufferers (Byrne & Gurdon, 2002; Lanza et al. 2000; NBAC, 1999; Stephenson, 2000). In the future, embryonic stem cells could potentially be used to produce not only replacement cells, but even entire replacement organs (Cibelli et al. 2001; Lanza et al. 2000).

A stem cell is a not yet fully differentiated cell, taken from an embryo, a fetus or a born human being, which possesses the ability to divide and develop in a specific way. Stem cells are capable of renewing themselves and of producing differentiated cells. They are therefore also in a position to regenerate tissue (Beier, 2002; Badura-Lotter, 2002). According to how far differentiation has progressed, a distinction is made between three different types of stem cell, namely *undifferentiated*, *embryonic* or *adult* stem cells.

Undifferentiated stem cells are at the first stage of embryonal development. They — like the fertilized egg cell itself — are *totipotent*, i.e. capable of developing into a complete organism (Beier, 2002; NIH, 2001). Totipotent cells can differentiate into extraembryonic tissue (such as the placenta), the embryo or any of the postembryonic tissue types or organs (NIH, 2001). In a uterus a human totipotent cell can develop into a complete individual, a human being (Beier, 2002). It is not known exactly how long these stem cells retain their totipotency. Various authors believe that the cells probably only retain this ability up to the two or four-cell stage (NCB, 2000). Others believe that even cells at the eight-cell stage could still be totipotent (Beier, 2002).

The second distinct stem cell type is the so-called embryonic stem cell (ES cell). These cells can be isolated from the inner cell mass of a blastocyst.[6] This stem cell type is no longer capable of developing the extraembryonic tissue crucial for the development of an embryo (Beier, 2002; NIH, 2001).[7] As a result, ES cells cannot develop into a complete human being (Beier, 2002; Wiestler & Brüstle, 2002). However, they can still develop into all the different types of tissue found in a human being. This characteristic is known as *pluripotency* (Beier, 2002; NIH, 2001). Two other types of pluripotent stem cell are embryonic germ cells (EG cells) and embryonal carcinoma cells (EC cells) (NBAC, 1999). The first of these, the EG cells, can be acquired in the laboratory from the forerunners of egg and sperm cells, the so-called primordial germ cells. EC cells are stem cells from the teratocarcinoma.

The third stem cell type, the *adult* stem cell, also known as the tissue-specific stem cell, consists of the stem cells from born human beings. Until recently it was assumed that this stem cell type could only differentiate into cell types of the tissue it itself belonged to (cf. Badura-Lotter, 2002; Wiestler & Brüstle, 2002). In recent years, however, it has been possible to observe differentiation of adult stem cells into cell types not included in the specific cell lines of the tissue they originated from (Beier, 2002; Badura-Lotter, 2002; Wiestler & Brüstle, 2002; see below).

In 1988 scientists succeeded for the first time ever in isolating human embryonic stem cells and reproducing them in cultures (Shamblott et al. 1998; Thomson et al. 1998). Thompson *et al.* managed to remove human ES cells from blastocysts, keep them alive and multiply them. This made them the first to manufacture human ES cell lines (Thomson et al. 1998). In the same year, scientists from the Johns Hopkins University in Baltimore were able to generate human EG cell lines from the primitive spermatoblasts of aborted fetuses (Shamblott et al. 1998). These successes meant the dawn of revolutionary prospects for the research field of tissue engineering (Denker, 1999; Heath, 2000; Lanza et al. 1999a). If mankind could gain information about the molecular mechanisms regulating the differentiation of human ES cells in a particular direction, then homogenous populations of numerous different cell types could be manufactured.

---

[6] A blastocyst comprises an external skin which later becomes the extraembryonal tissue, and an inner cell mass which later becomes the embryo (Rohwedel, 2001).

[7] According to Denker (2002), however, there is still no definitive proof that ES cells cannot be totipotent.

These in turn could then maybe be used for cell implantation in conjunction with certain defects. Maybe therapies could be developed for diseases which to date have no adequate treatment. Existing, unsatisfactory therapies could maybe also be improved (Perry, 2000), for example some cardiovascular diseases, cancer, diabetes or nervous disorders like Parkinson's disease. Maybe different cell types could even be produced in the laboratory as required, for example insulin-producing cells, dopamine-producing nerve cells or myocardial cells.[8] Maybe blood-producing stem cells could be manufactured and then used as an alternative to donor bone marrow cells in the treatment of patients whose bone marrow cannot (any longer) produce these cells itself. Hepatic cells generated in the laboratory could be used in the treatment of patients whose own livers are no longer capable of replacing damaged cells. And even the production of complete tissue types and organs could become possible (cf. Höfling, 2001; Lanza et al. 1999a).

Transplanting embryonic stem cells to a recipient organism might lead to rejection problems, however (Wiestler & Brüstle, 2002). After all, the ES cells would not be from the recipient. Present discussion focuses on three strategies to circumvent the different reactions of the recipient immune system (Heath, 2000; Prelle, 2001). The first strategy is to suppress such reactions with drugs. The second strategy is to manipulate the cells before implantation — for example, genetically — so that the recipient immune system could no longer recognize them as exogenous and trigger a rejection reaction (Curtis & Riehle, 2001; Heath, 2000; Lanza et al. 2000; Odorico et al. 2001). The third strategy is so-called 'therapeutic cloning'. The aim behind this strategy is to harvest endogenous ES cells which will not be subject to rejection reactions (Coors, 2002). It could be performed as follows: Firstly, the cell nucleus of a somatic cell from the recipient of the envisaged tissue or organ would be isolated and transferred — using the so-called 'cell nuclear transplantation technique' — to the plasma of an egg cell from which the cell nucleus had previously been removed. Inside this egg cell case, the highly-differentiated genetic program of the cell nucleus would then undergo extensive reprogramming. As a result, it would once more become totipotent (Beier,

---

[8] First therapeutic effects in connection with stem cell therapy for the treatment of Parkinson's disease were observed in rats. Dopamine-producing neurons were generated from ES cells and then transplanted in the animals (Kim et al. 2002).

2002). It would then develop into a blastocyst — in the same way as a naturally produced fertilized egg cell. From this the desired ES cells could then be harvested, after which the blastocyst would be destroyed (Rehmann-Sutter, 2002). The nuclei of the ES cells would have the same genetic material as the nuclei of the cells of the recipient of the envisaged tissue or organ and would thus not trigger any rejection reactions after implantation (Both, 2001; Rehmann-Sutter, 2002).

This cloning technique — to be distinguished from so-called 'reproductive cloning' (which aims at creating a complete new human being) — is known as 'therapeutic cloning' (Coors, 2002; Wolf, 2002). It is aimed not at reproduction, but rather at the acquisition of ES cells for therapeutic purposes. The use of *adult* stem cells represents an alternative to the use of *embryonic* stem cells (Bianco & Robey, 2001; Rohwedel, 2001; Strehl et al. 2002; Zuk et al. 2001). Compared to embryonic stem cells, adult stem cells do have limited differentiation potential (Beier, 2002; NIH, 2001; Wiestler & Brüstle, 2002). The *in vitro* acquisition of adult stem cells in sufficient numbers is also problematic to date (NIH, 2001; Wiestler & Brüstle, 2002).

And yet the advantage of using this type of cell is that every human being naturally possesses his own adult stem cells. Particular kinds of stem cell — especially from the bone marrow or adipose tissue — can be removed from a person requiring that type of tissue and be made to produce in large numbers without any great risk (Badura-Lotter, 2002). This also has the benefit that rejection reactions, so feared in connection with the use of allogenous embryonic stem cells, would not be a problem at all (Badura-Lotter, 2002). Adult stem cells have a further advantage over embryonic stem cells, namely that of having a presumed lower carcinogenic potential (Badura-Lotter, 2002). On top of all this, the number of reports about cases of so-called 'transdifferentiation', i.e. the differentiation of adult stem cells into cell types not associated with their own tissue-specific cell lines, is growing (Abkowitz, 2002; Badura-Lotter, 2002; Beier, 2002; Jiang et al. 2002; Rohwedel, 2001; Prelle, 2001; Kooy & Weiss, 2000; Watt & Hogan, 2000; Wiestler & Brüstle, 2002). The differentiation potential of adult stem cells is thus extremely likely to be much larger than has previously been assumed (Badura-Lotter, 2002; Wiestler & Brüstle, 2002). The transdifferentiation mechanisms are still largely unknown, however (NIH, 2001; Wiestler & Brüstle, 2002).

On the basis of the medical research, conclusive, definitive statements are impossible as to which of the two types of stem cell —
embryonic or adult — with all their advantages and disadvantages
is better suited to the production of replacement cells and tissue
(Badura-Lotter, 2002; CBBAS, 2001; Colman & Kind, 2000; NIH,
2001; Orkin & Morrison, 2002; Rohwedel, 2001; Wiestler & Brüstle,
2002).

5.2 Evaluation of the research field objectives

5.2.1 *Objectives*

Increasing the therapeutic options available

The first objective behind further development of the research field
of tissue engineering is to increase the therapeutic options currently
available for the treatment of tissue damage and organ failure (Fuchs
et al. 2001; Johnson, 2000; Nerem, 2000; Risbud, 2001). Against the
background of an aging population in the Western world this objective has a particular relevance, since tissue and organ damage
increase with age (Luyten et al. 2001; Sterkman & Riesle, 2000). The
increase in therapeutic options expected as a result of tissue engineering techniques can best be demonstrated by drawing direct com-
parisons to currently used conventional treatments of organ and tissue damage — namely 1) organ transplantation, 2) surgical
reconstruction with foreign tissue, 3) the use of artificial prostheses
and 4) the artificial administration of metabolic products (Pollok &
Vacanti, 1996). Advocates of further developments in tissue engineering often refer to these existing treatments when underlining the
contributions they expect the field to make.

1) Conventional organ transplantation

In the last few decades enormous progress has been made in the field
of conventional transplantation. Knowledge has vastly improved
regarding precise surgical procedures, as well as how to deal with
rejection of the implanted organ by the recipient organism. For some
time now, the primary difficulty facing the field of transplantation
medicine has therefore been not so much the transplantation itself,
but rather the acute shortage of transplantation 'material'. The short-

age of donor tissue and organs is becoming more and more acute with each passing year (Oduncu, 2000).[9]

This very serious problem is further exacerbated by that of how exactly to deal with rejection reactions (Fuchs et al. 2001). Up until now, immunosuppressive drugs have been used to suppress rejection. Patients have to take this medication permanently, however, meaning that they have to put up with a variety of severe side-effects all of the time.[10] Some rejection reactions displayed by a recipient immune system can render a donor organ useless.

Another problem is the huge cost of conventional organ transplantation (Black, 1997). Costs are incurred not only for surgery on the recipient, but also for surgery on the donor, long stays in hospital (in the case of living donors for two patients), as well as for transport of the organ. Suppressing the rejection reactions is also very expensive. Last but not least, the patients — recipient and donor in the case of a living donor — have the psychological cost to bear of being confronted with all the risks involved.

Compared to this conventional form of therapy, tissue engineering — provided it were to be developed further — could offer the following prospects: Firstly, this technique would require — in contrast to traditional organ transplantation requiring complete organs or tissue — just a small number of transplantable cells in order to grow the desired organ or tissue. Using stem cell technology, perhaps in the future even large numbers of different organs could be grown. Then there would always be a sufficient number of organs available for implantation in patients with different diseases. The severe organ shortage resulting from the current lack of donors would be alleviated.

Secondly, the risks involved in conventional transplantation — for example the risks of surgery for allogenous organ donors or the risk of the implant being rejected for the recipient — could be lessened or avoided altogether. The possibility of using autologous cells, such as adult stem cells, as breeding material for the organs would render all immunosuppression — crucial in cases of allotransplantation — superfluous, ruling out the concomitant negative side-effects (Kim & Vacanti, 1999).

---

[9] For European data, see: www.eurotransplant.nl; site visited August 1 2005.

[10] Examples being increased susceptibility to infection, impaired wound healing, increased risk of malignant tumors, as well as liver and/or kidney poisoning.

Thirdly, if use of tissue engineering technology were to mean the possibility of storing organs, patients would no longer have to wait for up to long periods of time — as is presently the case for organ transplantation — for a life-saving replacement organ. The required organs would be ready and waiting. They could be stored in close proximity to the transplantation site and could be organized to meet all kinds of criteria — for example organ size.[11]

Fourthly, the financial cost would most probably be lower (Langer & Vacanti, 1993). Removal of donor organs and emergency transportation of these organs to a recipient hospital would no longer be necessary. Treatment costs for patients waiting for organs would also disappear. Using tissue engineering, it may also become possible to save the money spent on life-long suppression of rejection reactions. And finally, the grief and skepticism which organ donation from deceased patients often arouses in their next-of-kin could be avoided.

2) Surgical reconstruction using foreign tissue

In the second traditional form of therapy — namely surgical reconstruction — use can be made of patient tissue, organs or parts of organs with similar characteristics to the defective tissue, organs or parts of organs. And yet they do not originate from the same cell type as the defective tissue they are replacing. Replacement tissue, organs or parts of organs are principally recipient-compatible, provided enough suitable material can be harvested. Parts of the large intestine can, for example, be used as replacement tissue for the esophagus or the bladder (Pollok & Vacanti, 1996).

The disadvantage of this method is that the implanted tissue cannot entirely replace the functions of the original tissue because it is not of exactly the same cell type. Sometimes a replacement organ does not function properly (Fuchs et al. 2001). There is also an increased chance of undesirable side-effects occurring (Atala, 1999). Examples of this would be calcification of the replacement tissue or cancerous growths (Langer & Vacanti, 1993). For patients — and, in the case of donated tissue or organs, also for donors — the complication risks are manifold (Pollok & Vacanti, 1996).

---

[11] In theory it would even be conceivable that a reserve supply of organs could be produced for every individual from his own cells, ideally at a young age. If an organ should fail, this reserve supply could then be tapped, with the risk of rejection reactions amounting to nil.

Using tissue engineering — following further development — all of these disadvantages could be avoided. Exact controls when growing tissue, organs or parts of organs would facilitate precise matching with the desired cell type, for example. A complete and functioning replacement for the original tissue could thus be produced. Complications such as impaired functioning of the implant or cancerous growths on the implanted tissue could be almost entirely avoided.

3) Artificial prostheses

The third conventional form of therapy, the utilization of artificial prostheses, involves non-biological materials such as metal or plastic. This form of therapy is used to replace parts of the body like joints, heart valves or eye lenses. It also encompasses the use of dialysis or plasmapheresis machines,[12] as well as the recent addition of artificial hearts.

Unfortunately this form of therapy also has its disadvantages (Fuchs et al. 2001; Sterkman & Riesle, 2000; Suh, 2000). The recipient is at risk of infection, for example. This may lead to loss of the implant. In addition, the synthetic materials used do not last forever (Chapekar, 2000). They lack the renewal skills characterizing living structures. Metal can corrode and degrade, sometimes leading to chronic irritation.

Tissue engineering would render various surgical interventions, such as the repeated implantation of artificial prostheses, superfluous. The chronic irritations sometimes occurring in conjunction with artificial prostheses could also be avoided. In contrast to artificial prostheses, biohybrid implants would have all the characteristics of living structures.

4) Artificial administration of metabolic products

The fourth traditional form of therapy, the artificial administration of metabolic products, is currently used in cases where a so-called endocrine organ is no longer functioning sufficiently. Endocrine organs essentially secrete hormones into the circulatory system. Examples of such organs are the pituitary gland, the thyroid gland or

---

[12] A plasmapheresis machine separates plasma from blood cells, for example in a blood sample. The blood cells — enriched with foreign plasma or saline solution — are subsequently reinfused.

the suprarenal gland. Patients are artificially administered with the hormones their organs are no longer producing, for example insulin. This usually occurs orally or by injection.

The disadvantage of this method is that the metabolic products have to be administered long-term. There is also a danger of the hormone balance becoming disturbed, with all the related negative consequences. The feedback given by a functioning organ is absent when hormones are administered artificially (Pollok & Vacanti, 1996).

If tissue engineering were to be developed further and implemented in clinical practice, maybe the permanent administration of hormones would cease to be necessary. By the same token, it would no longer be necessary to make readjustments to the hormone balance, a permanent requirement when metabolic products are administered artificially and a process unfortunately subject to error.

Advances in research

The second important objective behind the research field of tissue engineering — besides increasing the therapeutic options available — is advances in research (King & Patrick, 1998; Pedersen, 1999; Skalak et al. 1988). The practice of isolating cells and cultivating them outside the body dates back to the beginning of the 20th century (cf. Fell, 1972). It facilitates research into the way in which cells function *in vitro*. Isolated cell cultures have one big disadvantage, however. The specific cell behavior of isolated cells changes *in vitro*. It regresses. This phenomenon, whereby cells more or less develop backwards, is known as dedifferentiation. Due to this dedifferentiation taking place in isolated cells, the cell cultures available to date have only been of limited help to researchers investigating tissue and organ functions. Some tissue-typical behaviors cannot be simulated *in vitro*. In order to research the behavior of various living cells — for example their reaction to certain hormones, vitamins or drugs — 'functioning' tissue and organ cultures are required. Research on living organisms — without cultures at all — is not a good option either. In the living organism systemic reactions are often too complex (Fell, 1972, 8ff.).

Tissue engineering is aimed, amongst other things, at a better comprehension of the fundamental relationships between structure and function in normal tissue, as well as pathological tissue (Skalak et al. 1988). Tissue engineering technology promises to imitate *in vitro* the specific conditions of cells living *in vivo*, an option much called for

(Risbud, 2001). And this possibility of growing 'functioning' cell cultures in an artificial environment in turn promises various other prospects for research. A culture of 'functioning' pluripotent stem cells would be helpful, for example, in connection with research into the ways in which different drugs take effect, or into various environmental influences on the early embryo (Prelle, 2001). Pluripotent stem cells are similar to the cells of an embryo in its early stages of development (Rohwedel, 2001). The environment surrounding a cell culture could be 'furnished' to suit the research object in question. In this way tissue engineering might also be able to facilitate research into various new medications for adult humans. Maybe detailed tests and toxicological investigations could be performed on a whole range of different human cell cultures *in vitro* (NCB, 2000; Rohwedel, 2001). The insights gained in this way would probably be far more reliable, and they would be easier to transfer to human beings than the insights gained from animal experiments to date. In addition, tissue engineering could be helpful — through observation of the development of pluripotent stem cells similar to the cells of an embryo at the early stages of development — for research into the earliest events during the development of a human being at the cellular and molecular levels (Prelle, 2001; Rohwedel, 2001). Thus observation of the development of tissue and organs in an environment imitating nature could perhaps also become possible. This in turn could lead to a better understanding of cell differentiation mechanisms (Denker, 1999). This route could maybe also provide an answer to the origins of the different cell types, or to what causes the different cells to differentiate into certain tissue types or organs (Pedersen, 1999). This knowledge could in turn lead to the development of methods to control artificial triggering of the mechanism of cell differentiation.

In the course of further developments in the research field of tissue engineering it may in time become possible to examine more than living cell cultures. If it becomes possible to grow complex living tissue and organs, it will probably also become possible to perform research on them. This knowledge could then facilitate the early detection of certain tissue or organ-specific diseases, for example. In this way certain diseases could be treated much earlier than at present. The production of complex models for the investigation of pathogenic mechanisms would also be conceivable. And then tissue engineering would open up research into diseases which primarily affect the extracellular matrix, for example rheumatoid arthritis or arthrosis. Finally, the experiments performed on human tissue or organs, developed with the help of tissue engineering, would probably represent a suitable alternative to the experiments carried out on animals to date. Extensive expectations are pinned on the use of tissue engineering as an aid to research.

5.2.2 *Evaluation*

Increasing the therapeutic options available

Increasing the therapeutic options available has always been, and still is, the main objective of medical research. It is held in high esteem for two reasons. Firstly, a new and effective therapy can bring about improvements in the condition of patients. Secondly, it can — even when improvement is not possible — at least help to alleviate suffering. For both these reasons increasing the therapeutic options available does actually seem to be worth striving for. It contributes to the recovery and well-being of human beings — two esteemed phenomena.

A closer observation of different desirable phenomena uncovers the following distinction, however. On the one hand, there are some phenomena which are worth striving for in their own right. They include things like happiness or justice. Phenomena in this category possess a so-called intrinsic value. On the other hand, there are some phenomena which primarily serve as the means to other desirable ends, and which are thus indirectly worth striving for. They include tickets to the movies, bank bills and gift vouchers. This second type has a so-called extrinsic value.

Following this distinction, using tissue engineering to increase the therapeutic options available can be termed extrinsically valuable. It is a means to the desirable ends 'health' and 'well-being'. This renders it — and therefore the objective focused upon here — desirable.

Advances in research

At first sight, advances in research and the expansion of knowledge they inevitably bring with them, appear fundamentally desirable. Acquired knowledge *per se* can be both intrinsically and extrinsically valuable. For the person party to the knowledge it can represent a value in its own right — i.e. an intrinsic value. It can also provide a basis for potential new practical applications, rendering it extrinsically valuable, too. At first sight we could therefore conclude that this objective may be deemed desirable.

Taking a second look, however, the question arises of whether advances in research and the growth in knowledge they bring really are fundamentally desirable. Examined closely, increased knowledge can even, in certain circumstances, be capable of causing unhappiness. In Ancient times the Biblical sage Qoheleth wrote: "For in much wisdom is much grief: and he that increaseth knowledge increaseth sorrow." (Eccl. 1,18). Certain knowledge can *de facto* promote unhappiness.[13] But people attributing a loftier status to knowledge than happiness might say: "Better to be unhappy and knowledgeable than happy and unknowledgeable".

We may safely assume here, however, that the insights potentially to be gained from further developments in the research field of tissue engineering would not belong to the category of knowledge that could make people unhappy. These insights would comprise biological and biomedical advances in research — a deeper understanding of certain embryonic developmental processes, for example, or of the pathogenesis of certain diseases — and have been longed for by numerous researchers amid great expectations and scientific curiosity. Therefore this kind of knowledge, as well as its corresponding advances in research, can for now be deemed intrinsically valuable. In addition, there is a genuine chance that the insights resulting from advances in tissue engineering research could be helpful for the (fur-

---

[13] The following example illustrates how the acquisition of knowledge does not always have to be desirable. In the ongoing debate about prenatal diagnostics, the following view is often put forward in conjunction with Huntington's disease: Prenatal diagnostics should only be performed in cases where the prospective parents fundamentally agree in advance to a termination of the pregnancy should the diagnosis be positive. This example is not given in order to analyze the view itself. It is given because of the idea behind this view: A child has a right to be born without knowing that it is a carrier of Huntington's disease. It is not reasonable to expect a person to cope with this kind of information. A person living without the knowledge that he is disposed to a severe disease (like Huntington's) lives more freely and therefore more happily than with the knowledge that he has the disease and that it will probably surface around a certain age. People should be able to decide as adults whether or not to have themselves tested. In medical ethical discussions to date there has therefore been talk of a 'right not to know'. The mere existence of these contemplations — regarding the withholding of certain knowledge from certain people under certain circumstances — implies that the expansion of knowledge *per se* is not always a good thing, in contrast to the phenomena health, happiness or justice. Thus increased knowledge should not automatically be taken as equivalent to increased happiness or well-being.

ther) development of therapies for particular diseases and/or measures to prevent them. Of course, the extent to which this will actually be the case in the future ultimately remains open.

5.3 Contribution of the research field to realizing the objectives

5.3.1 *Increasing the therapeutic options available*

The question of whether further development of the research field of tissue engineering, as well as its application in medicine, would really contribute to realizing this objective cannot be answered with absolute certainty. It is true that tissue engineering is aimed, amongst other things, at the development of new effective therapies for a number of diseases and defects. And the comparison drawn above between tissue engineering and the four traditional forms of therapy — namely conventional organ transplantation, surgical reconstruction, the use of artificial prostheses and the artificial administration of metabolic products — really does indicate a potential increase in the scope of therapeutic possibilities. If this new research field were to be further developed, it would therefore be possible, at least in theory, for the application of tissue engineering technology to increase the therapeutic options available.

And yet the extent to which individual advances will actually occur necessarily remains open. A number of scientists, optimistic about future tissue engineering achievements, are placing their trust in the continued progress of stem cell technology, which they believe to be so promising. Whether and to what extent this technology will actually be able to fulfill the high expectations placed on it, however, depends on the fundamental and still unanswered question of whether the differentiation of stem cells can be precisely controlled (CBBAS, 2001; Lanza et al. 2000; Stock & Vacanti, 2001). Neither is it clear yet just how great the differentiation potential of the various human pluripotent stem cells is *in vitro* (Rohwedel, 2001). For example, we do not yet know whether isolated human ES cells have the same differentiation capacity as *in vitro* ES cells from mice (Rohwedel, 2001). A further problem is that of rejection reactions occurring following an allogenous transplantation of stem cells (CBBAS, 2001). And would acquisition of ES cells by therapeutic cloning — meaning the harvesting of recipient-compatible pluripotent stem cells — truly provide a satisfactory solution to the rejection problem? Or would it just open up a whole new can of worms? It is still uncertain, for example, whether the production of ES cell lines using this acquisition method would ever be efficient enough for application in clinical practice (Both, 2001; Colman & Kind, 2000; Rohwedel, 2001). If it proved to be not very efficient, then a large number of eggs would be required to produce just a single human ES cell line with success, and eggs are not available in limitless supply.[14]

Moreover, the cloning of mammals by transplanting cell nuclei from fully differentiated cells has so far not appeared to be very efficient (Moore, 2001; PHC, 2002). The majority of cloned animals have died early or suffered from various health problems (PHC, 2002), the causes of which have yet to be clearly identified. Searching for possible reasons, experts are currently discussing problems in connection with the reprogramming of the somatic cell nucleus, with imprinting, with mutations and with telomeres, amongst other things (Moore, 2001; PHC, 2002). If similar problems were to occur with the cloning of human beings as with the cloning of other mammals, this would definitely be fatal for possible human *reproductive* cloning. The problems under discussion could also have a negative effect on *therapeutic cloning*.[15] The reprogramming of the nucleus of a somatic cell for the purposes of therapeutic cloning could have such a negative effect on the differentiation potential of the stem cells to be harvested that the cells would no longer be capable of differentiating into different cell types as envisaged. And what about the potentially greater number of mutations in the cell nuclei of 'artificially produced' pluripotent stem cells compared to those emerging naturally (Both, 2001)? Compared to the latter, the former would, after all, be subjected to aggressive environmental influences for considerably longer. As a result of the advanced age of 'artificially produced' pluripotent stem cells, the telomeres (see 8.1.3) in their cell nuclei would probably be shorter than their natural equivalents (Both, 2001; but cf. Cibelli et al. 2002). How serious a problem would this be?

---

[14] With this in mind, the use of animal egg cells is currently being discussed. They are more widely available than human egg cells. Their use, however, would involve special problems and risks about which we do not yet know enough (Colman & Kind, 2000).

[15] It should not be taken for granted that problems surrounding reproductive cloning would also occur in conjunction with therapeutic cloning. The latter only requires intact blastocysts for the harvesting of ES cells and is not directed at the development of complete organisms (Lanza et al. 1999b).

Against the background of all the abovementioned problems, it is not possible to say at present whether therapeutic cloning could really contribute to the therapy of disease in the future (Both, 2001; Colman & Kind, 2000).[16]

In addition to all these unanswered questions in connection with therapeutic cloning, various other problems exist regarding stem cell technology. In many cases, for example, not enough is known about the precise factors and signals governing the differentiation of stem cells. In connection with the use of embryonic stem cells it is unclear how best to prevent differentiated tissue growth from still having ES cells. Such cells would harbor the risk of uncontrolled tumors (Both, 2001; Heath, 2000; Odorico et al. 2001). In connection with the use of adult stem cells, there is the question of just how substantial the ability of transdifferentiation would be (CBBAS, 2001). And how exactly can such stem cells be isolated and multiplied (Stock & Vacanti, 2001)?[17] The uncertain development of stem cell technology is, however, only one of many uncertainty factors affecting a prognosis of the extent to which the application of tissue engineering would really increase the range of therapeutic options available. It also remains uncertain whether in the future complete, complex, implantable organs could really be grown.

A multitude of problems is currently hindering the production of complete organs *de novo* in a purely artificial environment (Johnson, 2000). Research is still ongoing, for example, into the exact process of tissue and organ development, from the isolated starter cells up to full functioning capacity. Very little is known about the development process to date. This is partly due to the fact that we do not yet have sufficient information about the specific factors influencing the new formation of complex organs. These factors are only satisfactorily known for less complex tissue types like blood vessels and bones. Little is known about the generation of more complex organs like the kidneys. There is also little information available to date about how best to administer the different factors influencing new formation. We do not know the concentrations of the various molecules in the nutrient medium required to produce a certain effect, nor do we

---

[16] For further technical, medical and logistic problems surrounding therapeutic cloning, see Colman & Kind, 2000; Kind & Colman, 1999.

[17] For further issues and problems in connection with the use of adult stem cells for therapeutic purposes, see CBBAS, 2001.

know how long the starter cells must be exposed to them (Mooney & Mikos, 1999). Research is also being performed in the area of optimizing the supply of various nutrients to biohybrid tissue and organs (Risbud, 2001). Without an optimum supply of oxygen and nutrients to all the cells, no sizeable organ structures can be developed. And yet we do not know enough about the extent to which the tissue or organ in question could be furnished with a network of blood vessels before it is implanted (Curtis & Riehle, 2001; Fuchs et al. 2001; Griffith & Naughton, 2002; Terada et al. 2000). In the face of this vascularization problem, some hold the view that instead of producing complete complex organs *ex vivo* and implanting them, it would be more practical to concentrate on the renewal processes already existing *in vivo* and to substitute the missing components as needed (Stark et al. 2000a).

Many other problems of a more general nature also remain insufficiently solved, for example how to reverse the process of dedifferentiation, which begins in the starter cells as soon as they are isolated (Chapekar, 2000). Also being investigated are possible ways of avoiding rejection reactions following the implantation of biohybrid tissue. Allogenous starter cells — used for development when the patient does not have enough of his own intact cells — are fundamentally viewed by the recipient organism as hostile invaders. They often trigger hefty immune reactions which can lead to the destruction of implanted tissue. The risk of uncontrolled cell growth is another area under investigation. Researchers are trying to find out whether, and under what conditions, transplanted tissue will remain stable inside a living organism. Some researchers fear tumorous cell growth.

The research field of tissue engineering is still very new. And a whole range of difficult, as yet insufficiently explained problems remains to be solved (Curtis & Riehle, 2001; Chapekar, 2000). Nevertheless various scientists are already very hopeful that it will be possible to solve all these problems (Langer & Vacanti, 1999; Mooney & Mikos, 1999; Noishiki, 2001). Based on what has been achieved so far, they are assuming that the various technologies will continue to develop successfully over the years to come.

5.3.2 *Advances in research*

It is easier to answer the question of whether the research field of tissue engineering contributes to this objective than to the previous one. It seems probable that the application of different tissue engineering research techniques would be accompanied by an increase in knowledge. Because of the similarity between pluripotent stem cells and the cells of an embryo at the early stages of development (Pedersen, 1999; Rohwedel, 2001), the *in vitro* differentiation of ES cells could be used as a model system for research into the differentiation processes taking place within the cells of young embryos. Pluripotent stem cells could also be used for pharmacological and embryotoxicological research purposes. Of course, we cannot know how successful individual investigations with such model systems would actually be. A summarizing look at the other abovementioned examples (see 5.2.1) reveals that the new research field — provided it is further developed successfully — really would be capable of contributing to the expansion of knowledge in various medical areas. Here too, of course, we cannot yet know any details. It is also uncertain whether the insights gained would be substantial or whether they would lead to new therapies.

5.4 Ethical problems

5.4.1 *Responsible development and appropriate use*

Informed consent

Assuming for a moment that the practice of tissue engineering would develop to such an extent that at some stage it became possible to store all sorts of harvested cell samples in special cell banks until they were actually needed (cf. CBBAS, 2001; Moore, 2001; NCB, 2000; Vacanti & Vacanti, 2000),[18] then there would always be a sufficient number of starter cells available for tissue engineering purposes, be it for research or for therapy.

Before a cell sample could be stored for any purpose, however, including later use as starter cells for tissue engineering, the donor would have to be provided with sufficient information about the exact procedure and its consequences and then agree to it freely. In other words he would have to give his *informed consent* (Bennet, 2001;

---

[18] De Wert addresses the possibility of establishing individual cell banks. Isolated stem cells would be harvested at birth from blood in the umbilical cord and then stored for that individual (Wert, 2001b). Other authors are even discussing the possibility of off-the-shelf tissue engineering products (Johnson, 2000; Mooney & Mikos, 1999).

Erikson, 2001; HGC, 2002).[19] Obtaining the consent required for ethically justifiable storage and use of cell samples could prove difficult, however.

Ethical problems in this context concern the tests which the cell samples would have to undergo in order to be declared fit for use as starter cells in tissue engineering. Each potential allogenous cell sample would be subjected to different fundamental controls. In addition to viral tests, genetic tests would also be performed. The latter would provide information about whether the cell sample in question contained any detectable undesirable genetic defects. Hence these tests would also result in information about the genetic profile of the donor, information which could become more and more detailed as tests improve. These test results could be inopportune if genetic defects were to be discovered. Information about the existence of unfavorable genetic structures — which in the long term could maybe lead to a disease with no known prevention — could, for example, lead to depression and even suicidal tendencies in the donor (see below). It could also be disadvantageous for the donor if information about the existence of unfavorable genetic structures in his hereditary material were to fall into the wrong hands (see below). As a result, potential donors of starter cells would have to be informed in detail about the possible consequences of the tests prior to giving a cell sample, having it tested and having it stored.

However, giving donors extensive information regarding all the different tests, their potential results and all their possible consequences right down to the last detail could turn out to be extremely complicated. Hence the question arises of just how informed a donor would really need to be regarding the necessary tests. Would it be sufficient, for example, following an appropriate global information campaign, to obtain a general agreement from the cell sample donor as consent that his starter cells may be tested? This option would have the advantage that it would considerably simplify the informed consent procedure. It is debatable, however, whether a general agreement would be permissible in the face of the very complex material being agreed to. The view that individual consent would have to be obtained for each test performed is therefore also viable. This would

---

[19] If the donor of the cell sample were to be an embryo or fetus or small child, then the parents would have to give their informed consent to storage of the cell sample.

have the advantage that consent would be far more informed. The disadvantage would of course be its probable lengthiness in the face of so many special and detailed questions.

The following development could exacerbate the problem further. If, as assumed above, cell samples really could be stored in cell banks until needed, a great deal of time could elapse between their harvesting and their actual clinical application. In the face of the present rapidity of medical progress, however, it could well happen that in the interim storage period new tests would become available. Maybe these tests could be used to detect genetic defects in the cell samples which were not detectable when the cells went into storage.

With this scenario in mind, the issue of informed consent becomes a choice between two evils. *Either* the cell sample donor would have to give his general consent to all potential future tests. Then it would be difficult, if not impossible, to adhere to the prerequisite of informing the donor in advance and in detail about all the possible consequences. Who can give detailed information about tests which might become possible at a later date? *Or* the institute performing the tests would have to contact the donor prior to each new test in order to provide the relevant information and obtain the required consent. This would enable detailed information to be given about the new test, but it would considerably hinder the practicability of the informed consent procedure. Each donor would have to remain registered for his entire life, entailing huge administrative efforts and financial costs. Is it reasonable to expect a donor to maintain contact with the institute for the rest of his life? And what about cases in which a donor cannot be found, for whatever reason, and informed consent cannot be obtained?

One possible way of circumventing the aforementioned problems would be to wipe a cell sample clean of all factors characterizing it as belonging to a particular donor and to destroy all personal data. This would make it fundamentally impossible for cell banks to pass on test results to donors. If a donor were interested in a particular genetic diagnosis, he would still be able to have himself tested elsewhere. The advantage of this complete anonymity for cell samples would be that a general agreement from the donor, following information about use of the cells as starter cells for tissue engineering, would now be sufficient. The need to keep reobtaining consent for every single new test in the future would be rendered superfluous (Schröder & Williams, 2002). Anonymity of stored cells would also mean, however, that in cases where information might be discovered which could be useful to the donor — for example facilitating prevention of an imminent disease — it would be impossible for this information to be passed on. Before putting this anonymity into practice, it would have to be established for each envisaged cell sample application whether it would be sensible to maintain at least a roundabout way of linking the clinical and genetic donor data. If a link turned out to be essential — e.g. for particular research purposes — then the complete anonymity of cell samples would not be an option.

Overall, there are thus several important points regarding the problematic area of informed consent which are still open to discussion. They would need to be settled before an ethically justifiable practice of storing, testing and utilizing cell samples as starter material for tissue engineering could be developed.

Dealing with test results

Another problem could arise in dealing with the variety of information gained about the health of a donor in conjunction with cell sample testing. The following potential conflict exists regarding the tests performed to ascertain cell suitability. On the one hand, there would be an obligation *prima facie* to inform the donor of a cell sample about his test results. The donor would have a right to know (Häyry & Takala, 2001; Takala, 2001). The information would concern his own genetic constitution, after all. On the other hand, the donor would also have a fundamental right not to be informed (Bennet, 2001; Council of Europe, 1997; UNESCO, 1997). In certain cases the results could constitute a burden he could well do without.

Were all tests to be passed, a donated cell sample would be declared fit, and adhering to an obligation to inform would pose no problems. In cases where defects were detected for which successful therapies already existed, there would, generally speaking, also be no problem regarding an obligation to inform. In such cases the information would appear beneficial and thus clearly desirable. It would mean bad news, of course, for example the existence of genetic structures which could bring about a disease later in life (*late onset disease*). And yet, in the light of existing preventive measures for the looming disease, this news could only be advantageous to the cell sample donor. In principle there would be no reason not to fulfill an obligation to inform.

But what about a *prima facie* obligation to inform in cases where test results revealed a defect linked to a disease for which there was no adequate therapy to date? Should this obligation still be fulfilled in the full knowledge that, at the present time at least, the information would not benefit the donor and could even harm him? Test results could, for example, reveal a late onset disease for which preventive measures were yet to be found. The cell sample donor would probably get next to no benefit from receiving this information, and could possibly suffer badly as a result. The information might be helpful for family or career planning. Maybe the disease could be 'prepared for'. And yet it is unlikely that these benefits would outweigh the depression and anxiety which knowledge of a looming fatal disease would trigger. In the course of rapidly increasing expertise in the field of genetics, the range of diagnosable genetic defects causing late onset diseases would probably increase just as rapidly. Since there is no reason to assume that this would go hand in hand with a corresponding rise in the number of new therapies, the conflict of just how to react in such cases with regard to an obligation to inform could in time occur more and more frequently.

An ethically justifiable decision to inform donors about certain test results would therefore have to include considerations like a cost/benefit analysis of receiving such information. But who should be entitled to judge the benefits ensuing from a problematic piece of news? The institute carrying out the tests and thus having access to the results? Or should the donor himself have the right to decide whether he wants to know or not? One possible solution could be to discuss with the donor in advance — during the obtaining of his informed consent — which results he would like to be informed of, and which should be kept from him. This would mean the very practical problem, however, of making the already complex procedure for obtaining informed consent even more complicated. There would also be the problem of which defects and diseases the donor should be required to decide about. And should test results be revealed for defects not included on the list as seen by the donor? This could happen, for example if a particular defect could not be tested for at the time the donor signed the papers, but then became diagnosable at a later date due to advances in genetic research. And what would the correct behavior be regarding defects linked to diseases which could not be prevented at the time the donor signed, and which he therefore wished not to know about, but which later became treatable as a result of new medical advances?

One way of avoiding these problems has already been mentioned, namely to wipe cell samples clean of all factors identifying the donor and to destroy all personal data. This would relieve cell banks of repeated confrontation with the problem of how to behave regarding their obligation to inform every single time a new test became available which at the time a donor signed was not available. Here too, however, anonymity of cell samples would mean not being able to contact a donor if information in his own best interests came to light.

Data protection

In our Information Age, it seems to be becoming increasingly difficult to provide adequate guarantees for either privacy or data protection (Brin, 1998; Sykes, 1999; Whitaker, 1999). It may therefore not be possible to guarantee the security of digitally stored test results from cell samples intended for banking as potential starter cells for tissue engineering. For the donors of these cell samples, this could lead to problems. In time, testing of cell samples could reveal the genetic profiles of the donors. If this information were to fall into the wrong hands, both the donors themselves and their families would be at risk of discrimination, for example at work, during job applications or when taking out health insurance. The following three groups would be particularly interested in test results which reveal the genetic profiles of certain individuals: employers, insurance companies, and the law.

Employers strive to employ people with perfect health wherever possible. For this reason every potential employee has to undergo a medical check-up.[20] This examination is supposed to reveal qualities and defects directly associated with the envisaged workplace. The big advantage of test results from genetic diagnoses would be their inclusion of at least some information about a job applicant's health in the future. Due to growth in genetic expertise and the development of more precise genetic testing methods, the scope and reliability of this information will probably continue to increase. Bearing this in mind, it would come as no surprise if employers were to attempt to gain access to cell bank databases in the future.

---

[20] These check-ups are, of course, also performed for the protection of employees. Somebody found to be suffering from bronchitis, for example, should not regularly be made to work with mortar.

The second group, that of the insurance companies, strives to ascertain the health risks of potential policy holders as precisely as possible. For this reason they would definitely be interested in gaining access to genetic profiles. A profile would provide them with precisely the information they require about the future health of a potential policy holder in order to calculate, more or less, his exact risk. They too could thus endeavor to gain access to cell bank databases in the future.

The law, the last of the three groups, could be interested in various test results due to the fact that genetic profiles could help to identify selected suspects much more quickly. It would be easy to prove the guilt or innocence of certain individuals with access to their genetic make-up.

The key issue here — namely how potential misuse of test results could be prevented — can only be decided by addressing the difficulty of how to guarantee data security in the cell banks of the future. Once again, this could be achieved by wiping cell samples clean of all factors identifying the donors. By destroying all data which could identify a donor, discrimination would be ruled out from the start. But of course, once again, information coming to light which could be of benefit to a donor could no longer be passed on.

A thorough discussion about security measures would therefore have to take place prior to the setting up of databases to store results from diagnostic tests on cell samples. In this discussion, decisions would have to be reached as to how exactly future genetic data would be stored, and who would have access to this information.[21]

5.4.2 Problems intrinsically linked with the technology

Embryo protection

In theory, different cell types could be used as starter cells in tissue engineering, namely totipotent, pluripotent and adult stem cells, as well as fully differentiated cells. As already mentioned above, individual isolated totipotent stem cells are fundamentally capable, in the right conditions, of growing into complete human beings. One of the things they would require to do this — removed as they are from

---

[21] Problems surrounding the confidentiality of personal genetic data are already being discussed in connection with currently existing DNA banks and biobanks (Hansson, 2001; HGC, 2000 & 2002; Schröder & Williams, 2002).

their original cell group — would be an artificial *zona pelucida* to re-encase them. The resulting formation would then have to be implanted in a uterus. This kind of experiment has yet to appear in the literature, however.

Regardless of the fact that this ability of totipotent cells to develop into a complete human being must remain purely theoretical for now, some authors are already equating them with embryos (WICDA, 1991). Accordingly, totipotent stem cells are being defined as formations which, under the right circumstances, would be capable of developing into complete organisms. This equation gives rise to the following problem, however: Using totipotent cells, or 'embryos', to grow tissue or complete organs would lead to their sure destruction. Encouraging stem cells to grow into a particular tissue type or organ would necessarily prevent them from developing into a complete human being.[22] Using totipotent stem cells to grow tissue or complete organs would therefore be ethically problematic, or at least for those people who believe an embryo to be worthy of full protection from the very first stage of its development.

A similar problem is being discussed in conjunction with embryonic stem cells (ES cells) (cf. Wert, 2001a). According to our present knowledge, isolated ES cells have lost their totipotency — with cell differentiation occurring by the 8-cell stage — and yet it is at least theoretically possible that ES cells could grow into complete organisms, too. It is conceivable, for example, that these cells could be placed inside an empty blastocyst and left to develop (cf. Wert, 2001a). In this case ES cells could also be viewed as embryos. This would mean the same ethical problems for pluripotent cells as for totipotent cells, or at least for those people believing an embryo to be worthy of full protection from the very first stage of its development.

Most authors do not share this view that ES cells can be equated with embryos. In their view, this equation requires the concept of potentiality to be stretched unacceptably far. In theory it is possible to imagine ES cells developing into complete organisms. And yet because the differentiation potential of this stem cell type is significantly lower than that of totipotent stem cells, both the extent and the type of artificial interventions necessary for a complete organism to form would essentially differ from those in totipotent stem cells.

---

[22] In addition, the cell cluster remaining after the totipotent cells had been removed for breeding would possibly be damaged or destroyed, too.

The same is true for the difficulties which could occur using ES cells. The use of ES cells, in contrast to the use of totipotent stem cells, would firstly require the preparation of a sufficiently large cell culture. Then an empty blastocyst would have to be procured to encase the prepared ES cell mass. However, an empty blastocyst can only be obtained by removing the inner cell mass from an intact blastocyst. And this very act would be immoral in the eyes of those who believe that embryos are worthy of full protection from the start. Here too, we cannot know whether the theoretical possibility of developing a manipulated blastocyst into a complete organism could ever be achieved *de facto*.[23]

In the light of all these difficulties surrounding the use of ES cells to grow complete organisms, equating ES cells with embryos — and thus granting them an embryo-like status — would appear far-fetched, not to mention problematic. In addition, it would stretch the concept of potentiality so far that it would make the finding of convincing objections difficult, should somatic cells likewise be granted an embryo-like status. After all, complete animal organisms have already been created from animal somatic cells using the cloning method. And a corresponding achievement with human somatic cells in the future is not inconceivable. And yet attributing an embryo-like status to somatic cells would be extremely counter-intuitive, if not grotesque. In this analysis ES cells will therefore *not* be equated with embryos. In contrast to totipotent cells, where equation with an embryo seems to be at least debatable, ES cells are firmly *not* attributed with an embryo-like moral status.

This means that the ethical problems surrounding the use of pluripotent cells — in contrast to the use of totipotent cells — are not embedded in the characteristics of the cell type itself. It is far more the harvesting of pluripotent stem cells that poses the ethical problems. Four acquisition methods can currently be distinguished (cf. AAAS & ICS, 1999; NBAC 1999): 1) Primordial germ cells are taken from miscarried or aborted fetuses. These cells are the forerunners of egg and sperm cells. Following induced or spontaneous abortion they are isolated from the fetus and further developed in cultures to form embryonic germ cells (EG cells). 2) Embryonic stem cells (ES cells) are taken from blastocysts which are left over following in vitro

---

[23] From an ethical viewpoint an experiment of this nature would be highly problematic because of the great risks it would involve for the future child.

fertilization treatment (IVF). After about four or five days, during which several cell divisions occur, a fertilized egg cell reaches the blastocyst stage. Within roughly the next three days ES cells can then be isolated from the inner cell mass of the blastocyst (the embryoblast). As a result, the blastocyst is destroyed. 3) ES cells are taken from blastocysts which have been especially created for this purpose using IVF. The embryos resulting from the IVF procedure in this case are — in contrast to method no. 2) — used deliberately and exclusively for the acquisition of ES cells. They are not left over from fertility treatment. 4) ES cells are taken from blastocysts which have been especially created for this purpose using the cloning technique of cell nuclear transplantation ('therapeutic cloning').

A closer look at the ethical issues and potential problems surrounding these four methods of harvesting pluripotent stem cells reveals that they increase the further one progresses down the list. In the *first* method the acquisition of pluripotent stem cells does not involve destroying unborn life. The fetuses used are already dead. The use of dead fetuses purely as a means to an end could be considered problematic, however. A fetal corpse is instrumentalized for the purpose of acquiring coveted pluripotent stem cells. The *second* method involves not only the instrumentalization of an embryo, but also its calculated destruction, brought about unavoidably as a consequence of removing pluripotent cells from the embryoblast. The problem of instrumentalization occurs even more radically in the *third* method. Here it is not existing embryos, but embryos created especially for this purpose, which are used for the acquisition. A momentous difference between this method and the second one is that here the destruction of the embryo is intended all along (NBAC, 1999). In the *fourth and last* method, not only the fact that embryos are being created and then destroyed again for the sole purpose of stem cell acquisition is ethically problematic; so too is the method employed to create the embryos, namely cell nucleus transportation.[24]

All of the ethical problems listed in connection with the peculiarity of totipotent stem cells and the various possible ways of harvesting pluripotent stem cells stand opposed to the potential benefits —

---

[24] Some authors maintain, for example, that therapeutic cloning would open the floodgates to ethically problematic reproductive cloning (cf. Wert, 2001b; Lanza et al. 2000).

in the sense of improved health or alleviated suffering for patients —
which utilization of these stem cells in the production of replacement
tissue and organs could entail. Before deciding whether the use of
one or both of these stem cell types would be ethically justifiable at
all, and if so using which acquisition method, the listed ethical problems therefore have to be weighted. If, following this evaluation, certain ethical problems appear non-surmountable and too serious, then
the cell type in question should not be used and/or the acquisition
method in question not be pursued.

Precise weighting of the ethical problems listed is affected by
whether, and if so to what extent, an embryo is considered worthy of
protection. If, for example, an embryo were not considered worthy of
protection at all, then the ethical problems of instrumentalization and
destruction would vanish. The views which exist with regard to
embryo protection can be divided into conceptionalist and non-conceptionalist views.

According to the *conceptionalist* view, from the moment of its conception a developing embryo is equally worthy of protection as a
completely formed human being. This view is currently held by the
Roman Catholic Church, for example. In its instruction *Donum Vitae*,
which appeared in 1987, it declares that every human creature
demands without reservation the same esteem from the first moment
of its existence — i.e. the moment the zygote forms — as all human
beings are fundamentally morally entitled to. From the moment of
its fertilization a human creature must be treated like a person. It is
acknowledged as having the rights of a person from this moment
onwards. This particularly includes the sacrosanct right of every
human being to live (CvdG, 1987). This moral view stems from
numerous passages in the Holy Scriptures clearly illustrating God's
commitment to mankind from the beginning of time. In these passages it is God who initiates human pregnancy (Gen 29, 31; Gen 30,
22; Gen 49, 25; Ruth 4, 13). The same thing is maintained by the
author of Psalm 139 and by the Prophet Job: "Thine hands have
made me and fashioned me together round about; yet thou dost
destroy me. Remember, I beseech thee, that thou hast made me as the
clay; and wilt thou bring me into dust again?" (Job 10, 8f). Both speak
of God's involvement with man. Each individual human life —
according to the view of the Catholic Church — is desired by God.
The uniqueness of the relationship between man and God renders
each human life intrinsically valuable. It is not man's place to put an

end to human life (see, too, the Fifth of the Ten Commandments: 'Thou shalt not kill' (Ex 20,13)).

The conceptionalist view does permit the idea of conception being a drawn-out process. The process finishes with the establishment of a new genome. From this point onwards a new embryo worthy of full protection exists (Schockenhoff, 2001). In the light of new medical developments, 'conceptionalism' is no longer really a suitable term. Embryos can now be created without conception having to take place at all, e.g. using the techniques of blastomere separation or cell nuclear transplantation. Accordingly, this analysis will regard conceptionalism as the view that every embryo is worthy of full protection. The complex concept of the embryo itself is not problematized any further within this framework.[25]

Regarding starter cells for tissue engineering, use of totipotent stem cells *per se* and employment of the last three of the cited methods for acquiring ES cells are ethically unacceptable according to the conceptionalist view, due to the fact that embryos are destroyed in the process. Embryos are equally worthy of protection as fully developed human beings. The destructive use of embryos for research or therapeutic purposes would be just as ethically unacceptable, according to this view, as the killing of a fully developed human being for the sole reason that his corpse could be useful to another person. By contrast, the use of embryonic germ cells (EG cells) as starter cells for tissue engineering could be ethically justifiable for conceptionalists under certain circumstances. These cells would be harvested from aborted, thus already dead fetuses, which were not destroyed for the purpose of acquiring EG cells. However, there could be reservations about the ethical permissibility of using and thus instrumentalizing fetal corpses. Just as with the medical utilization of adult human corpses, here too a procedure of informed consent would have to be drawn up for the use of fetal tissue. In addition, measures would have to be taken to prevent cases where pregnancies are initiated and then terminated again for the sole purpose of harvesting EG cells. Overall though, for advocates of the conceptionalist viewpoint there is some scope for discussion regarding the suitability of EG cells as starter cells for tissue engineering.

---

[25] As mentioned earlier, in this analysis totipotent cells are regarded as embryos, ES cells are not.

According to the *non-conceptionalist* view, the degree to which an embryo is worthy of protection depends on its stage of development. At the beginning of its existence it is hardly worthy of protection, or even not worthy of protection at all. As the embryo grows, it becomes increasingly worthy of protection — either gradually or discontinuously, depending on the particular view. Thus the further the stage of development reached by the embryo, the worthier it is of protection. According to the non-conceptionalist view, there are moments or phases during ontogenesis which are morally so significant that they render a developing human being worthier of protection as a result. Examples would include implantation of the embryo in the wall of the uterus, completion of embryogenesis, the development of the nervous system, the ability to survive outside the mother, birth itself and the development of consciousness. According to non-conceptionalists, only a late fetus or even a born human being is worthy of full protection. The spectrum of protection which non-conceptionalist views can cover — from absence to total presence — provides a certain amount of scope as to what is still permissible or no longer permissible treatment of an embryo at a certain stage of its development.

The views of one important subgroup of non-conceptionalists regarding the embryo protection are based on neo-Lockean notions about the concept of person. These notions historically stem from the theory of person put forward by the English philosopher John Locke (1632-1704). In his view a person is a:

> "[...] conscious thinking thing (whatever substance made up of, whether spiritual or material, simple or compounded, it matters not) which is sensible, or conscious of pleasure and pain, capable of happiness or misery, and so is concerned for itself, as far as that consciousness extends." (Locke, 1690, 62).[26]

According to Locke's definition, the existence of *consciousness* is a prerequisite *sine qua non* for being a person. Locke's concept of consciousness is not unambiguous, however. And more seriously: Locke omitted to clarify whether in his view consciousness is one prerequi-

---

[26] Elsewhere he defines the person as "[..] a thinking intelligent being, that has reason and reflection, and can consider itself as itself, the same thinking thing in different times and places; which it does only by that consciousness which is inseparable from thinking, and as it seems to me essential to it: it being impossible for anyone to perceive, without perceiving that he does perceive." (Locke, 1690, 55).

site among many or in itself a sufficient prerequisite for being a person. The consequence of this omission is that over the years many different interpretations and modifications of his idea of consciousness as a prerequisite for being a person have emerged.

Today many authors — especially from the English-speaking world — have settled on the idea of viewing person as an entity which has at least a rudimentary kind of consciousness (Lizza, 1993; Warren, 1997). And yet most of these authors vary in opinion as to how the idea progresses beyond the mere possession of consciousness. They all propose individual characteristics and abilities which on their own or in combination supposedly constitute a person. Some of the more important are listed here (Tooley, 1983, 90f). They represent prerequisites for being a person in addition to the mere possession of consciousness:

- The ability to experience joy and suffering;
- The ability to have wishes;
- The ability to remember things past;
- The ability to have expectations about the future;
- The ability to perceive time;
- The characteristic of being an uninterrupted, conscious self, a subject, separate from one's mental states;
- The ability to be self-aware;
- The ability to have intentional states of consciousness;
- The ability to form arguments;
- The ability to solve problems;
- The characteristic of being autonomous;
- The ability to use a language;
- The ability to interact with others in a social manner.

In the course of time a multitude of neo-Lockean theories about person have emerged. And yet they all have one thing in common, namely that the status of person is not attributed to a human being until relatively far into his ontogenetic development.

The vast majority of authors regard this status as a necessary prerequisite for protection. This means that we can assume that the majority of supporters of neo-Lockean ideas about person would give an affirmative answer to the question about the ethical justifiability of using embryos *in vitro* to harvest stem cells.[27] According to

---

[27] Other authors believe that potential persons have the same moral status and are thus equally worthy of protection as actual persons (Reichlin, 1997; Vedder, 1993).

these authors, the moment during ontogenesis from which a developing human being is deemed worthy of full protection is definitely not before or during the developmental stages in which totipotent or pluripotent stem cells can be harvested. According to some authors, this moment is not even reached until some time after the birth (Singer & Wells, 1985). According to the non-conceptionalist view, an embryo *in vitro* is therefore either not worthy of protection at all (Hartogh, 1993; Harris, 1985; Singer & Dawson, 1990) or only relatively — i.e. less worthy than an adult (Wert, 1989; Kuitert, 1991; Reinders, 1993; Zoloth, 2000).[28] By contrast, the *conceptionalist* view believes an embryo *in vitro* to be equally worthy of protection as an adult (Eijk, 1997; Jochemsen, 1989; Kreeft, 1990; Pellegrino, 2000).

Taking these two views on embryo protection side by side, at first sight the conceptionalist view seems less convincing. Purely intuitively, an adult human being is deemed worthier of protection than, say, a fertilized egg cell. In an emergency situation, for example a hospital in flames, one would probably tend to rescue grown patients before rescuing frozen embryos. The ethical relevance of such intuitive judgements and subjective preferences is doubtful, however. In an emergency situation one would also tend to rescue a family member before rescuing a stranger. And yet this does not automatically mean that a stranger is less worthy of protection *from an ethical standpoint* than a family member. Regarding the attribute of being worthy of protection, this analysis will therefore concentrate not on emotional judgements but on ethical arguments.

As already mentioned above, various existing analyses of the problems surrounding embryo protection regularly employ both the concept of person and the concept of moral status (Juengst & Fossel, 2000; Meyer & Nelson, 2001; NBAC, 1999; NCB, 2000; Warren, 1997).[29] Instead of the terms 'person' and 'moral status' the author favors the term 'worthiness of protection'. The reason for this is that the term 'worthiness of protection' appears to the author to be considerably more explicit and precise than the other two terms. He

---

[28] The opinion that an embryo *in vitro* is not worthy of protection would not, however, automatically imply that all manner of activities with such embryos would be ethically permissible. These embryos could be attributed a symbolic value, for example (Hartogh, 1993).

[29] In addition — especially in the German debate — analyses contain terms such as 'being human', 'right to live', 'human right', 'protection of life' and 'human dignity' (Brüske, 2001; Höfling, 2001; Schockenhoff, 2001).

believes the terms 'person' and 'moral status' to be too broad and thus too vague (cf. Gordijn, 1999).

Three ethical arguments can be called on to support the view that embryos should be equally worthy of protection as adults: (1) the *reductio ad absurdum* argument, (2) the defense of the weak argument, and (3) the caution argument.

Argument 1 (*reductio ad absurdum*): Non-conceptionalist views assume that the attribute of being worthy of protection is linked to the possession of certain characteristics — e.g. consciousness, a certain degree of independence, particular interests or particular cognitive abilities — which an early embryo cannot possess, or at most can barely possess. It acquires them over the course of time, achieving in the process — whether gradually or suddenly — a new level of protection. To be consistent, however, this would mean that individuals who lost these characteristics would also have to forfeit their protection. Yet in turn this would mean that individuals in a coma, for example, or depressive individuals who due to their depression have few to no interests, or mentally disabled individuals would necessarily cease to be worthy of protection. This consequence is refuted by the moral intention *common sense*, however. Which means that the two non-conceptionalist views lead to absurd consequences (*reductio ad absurdum*). As a result, both must be rejected.

Argument 2 (defense of the weak): In the human community unborn human beings are the weakest of the weak. They cannot even impart their own interests. For this reason society should take great care not to subject this group to any procedures which it would not consider ethically viable in stronger groups. The two non-conceptionalist views permit such treatment, however. As a result, both must be rejected.

Argument 3 (caution): As long as there are no compelling arguments for attributing an embryo no or only little protection, care must be taken to treat it as if it were worthy of the full protection of an adult human being. Remaining consistent, embryos should thus not be subjected to any procedures which would not be ethically justifiable in adult human beings. Here the rule of tutiorism prevails: *idem est in moralibus facere et exponere se periculo faciendi* (from an ethical point of view, committing an act and putting oneself in danger of committing it have the same status). Transferred to the case in hand, this rule means: because it is not clear whether and to what extent embryos are worthy of protection, the instrumentalization of embryos should, for reasons of caution, be evaluated as if it were clearly immoral. It could turn out that embryos are entitled to full protection. And it would be immoral to put oneself in danger of violating this entitlement.

As a consequence of the above analysis of embryo protection, in summary it therefore seems ethically indicated not to use totipotent cells as starter cells for the production of replacement tissue and organs. As far as the use of pluripotent cells is concerned, the first of the four currently possible acquisition methods, namely the harvesting of EG cells from the primordial germ cells of already dead fetuses, is to be favored.

Various fears have been put forward in connection with the general use of fetal tissue, though. For example there is a fear that the practice of using dead fetuses for the acquisition of EG cells could lead to systematic abortions aimed at precisely the harvesting of these stem cells. It could also render medicine dependent on abortion (Boer, 1999; King & Patrick, 1998; NBAC, 1999; NBC, 2000). These and other fears should be taken seriously. If a decision is taken in favor of using EG cells harvested from the primordial germ cells of dead fetuses, then at the same time it should be ensured that all decisions to abort are made independently of any possibility of the fetal tissue being made available to the medical profession for the purpose of harvesting the EG cells within it (NBAC, 1999; NBC, 2000).

With the above ethical analysis in mind, research projects should be welcomed which attempt to use *adult stem cells* and *fully differentiated cell types* for production (cf. Kass, 2001). Neither use of these two cell types *per se* nor their acquisition involve the ethically problematic instrumentalization and destruction of embryos. Maybe in the future it will become technically possible to reprogram fully differentiated cells and turn back their genetic clock to the stage of pluripotency (cf. Beier, 2002; Lanza et al. 2000; NCB, 2000; Rohwedel, 2001). This would make pluripotent cells available without the need for embryos or fetuses. The ethical problems surrounding the destruction and instrumentalization of embryos would thus be circumvented.[30]

---

[30] In order for this option to be developed, more detailed research would most likely be required into the way in which a denucleated egg cell reprograms a somatic cell nucleus. The factors responsible for the reprogramming of an egg cell would have to be identified and then produced in the laboratory for use in the reprogramming of differentiated cells (Prelle, 2001). Although this phenomenon can be observed in other

5.4.3 Undesirable effects in the longer term

Enhancement potential of tissue engineering

Let us assume for a moment that tissue engineering were already as successfully developed as various current advocates of the research field are predicting will happen. All scientific problems connected with tissue engineering have been solved, and both the production and utilization of tissue and organs grown in the laboratory are now possible. This would mean the additional option of swapping tissue and organs, which for whatever reason are not 'ideal', for better, maybe even 'ideal' replacement tissue and organs free of faults. This would facilitate not only the possible elimination of 'faults' like a crooked nose or an impure skin; all kinds of wish could be fulfilled, like a stunning appearance or an extraordinarily strong and robust body. In so doing, tissue engineering would be providing not only *restitutio ad integrum* (restitution of the integral body and its functions), but also an improvement in human constitution beyond the purely curative (Black, 1997). The two traditional areas of medicine, namely 'healing' and 'prevention', would be extended to include a third area, 'enhancement'.[31]

Yet would this extension of tissue engineering to include human enhancement be desirable from an ethical point of view? At first sight the principle of beneficence could be used as an argument in defense of such an extension. This principle states that we should fundamentally strive to increase human well-being as much as possible. The question is, however, whether attempts to fulfill all kinds of optimization wish with the help of medicine would increase human well-being. It is just as conceivable that the enormous range of — possibly illusory — ways of enhancing human beings would open up people's eyes to just how 'imperfect' they really are. In addition, in the face of the apparently endless possibilities for improvement, the wishes of human beings would know no boundaries. Extending the field of tissue engineering to human enhancement could therefore, *summa summarum*, bring about more discontentment than before. It would not automatically signify an increase in human well-being.

---

species, it might be necessary to perform cloning experiments with human cells. And this in turn would involve the destruction of embryos (Wert, 2001a & 2001b).

[31] It is not possible within the framework of this book to go into the difficulty of where to draw the line between human therapy and human enhancement (see Lenk, 2002).

Furthermore, many human optimization wishes could potentially be treated more adequately with means other than purely medical ones. Underlying many wishes for optimization are problems (e.g. insecurity, frustration, discontentment) which could possibly be solved just as well or even better using psychotherapeutic, sociological, political, spiritual or philosophical means. Emphasizing the role of tissue engineering as a means of fulfilling all kinds of wish could possibly lead to an undesirable medicalization of the problems behind the wishes.

Finally, in the face of shortages in the health sector, as well as the uneven distribution of means worldwide, it is debatable whether medicine providing treatments on request, beyond the curative and preventive, would really be justifiable.

These critical observations make it impossible to form a clear ethical evaluation of the enhancement potential of tissue engineering. On the one hand, the seemingly attractive enhancement potential of tissue engineering is tempting; on the other hand, it is doubtful whether extending tissue engineering to include human enhancement would actually be desirable.

Attitudes towards the body

Further successes in the technical and scientific development of the research field of tissue engineering could lead to confusions in terminology and changes of attitude towards the body. For a long time the concept of body as used in medicine was unproblematic: 'the body' was everything inside the skin encasing an organism. The skin formed a clear boundary between the body and its surroundings. Everything outside this case unmistakably no longer belonged to the body.

This concept of the body has recently become confused in the light of various medical achievements. The new discipline of organ transplantation, for example, has facilitated the implantation of 'subparts' in the body which were previously located outside the body. The same has happened with artificial prostheses. Now, does an implanted organ or prosthesis become part of the body on implantation or does it remain foreign to the body? Equally unclear is the situation regarding devices which are connected to the body externally in order to assume essential physical functions, for example a dialysis machine or a heart-lung machine. In such cases it is not easy to say precisely what constitutes the 'body'.

It is to be expected that further developments in the field of tissue engineering would make this confusion concerning the concept of body even more extreme. What category would an organ belong to grown from a cell sample taken from the recipient's own body — meaning that it could be termed 'endogenous' — but developed outside the body and then implanted — meaning that it could just as easily be termed 'exogenous'? This would be exacerbated further by the fact that tissue and organs developed in the laboratory would probably in time cease to be distinguishable from their endogenous equivalents in appearance and function. Under the influence of tissue engineering the difference between 'natural' bodies — without any interventions of the type described — and 'manipulated' bodies — containing artificial subparts — would become increasingly blurred. In time it may even become non-existent.

Besides confusion regarding the concept of body, new medical options — for example in the area of transplantation medicine — have for some time now also been leading to new attitudes towards the body. Firstly, the various new therapeutic options available are increasingly giving the impression that the body is a whole, made up of many different components. Physical development, physical functions and specific physical characteristics are appearing less and less fixed by nature and to be accepted without change, and more and more controllable. It is believed that good function can be achieved by regularly replacing any defective parts. This changing attitude is increasingly encouraging an image of the body as a product of technology, equivalent to a machine.[32]

Secondly, a process of commercialization and commodification can be observed regarding the body (Andrews & Nelkin, 2001; Kimbrell, 1993): The body and all its subparts are increasingly becoming tradable goods. Cells, tissue and organs, as well as the 'borrowing' of a uterus have all become tradable and purchasable. Not only egg cells and sperm, but also hair, blood, umbilical cords, placentas and foreskins are increasingly becoming part of the economy surrounding the human body. Scientists and biotechnological companies are attempting to patent genes. Embryos and brain-dead human beings are being viewed as sources of replacement organs and tissue. The body

[32] The progress of reproduction medicine has contributed to this development. It implies that the development of the body is something which is increasingly determined by human intervention. Maybe in the course of this development the concept of a natural given body will lose its significance altogether.

is being treated almost like the inanimate material of a machine. In the process, the human being seems to be becoming increasingly de-hallowed and de-mystified (Andrews & Nelkin, 2001; Kimbrell, 1993).

Progress in the research field of tissue engineering could accelerate this change in attitudes towards the body. With the help of tissue engineering complete warehouses of replacement cells, tissue and organs could be set up, from which people could help themselves whenever they needed anything. The commercialization and de-hallowing of the human body and all its subparts could be spurred on further by this development.

Yet would accelerated confusion of the concept of 'body' and changing attitudes towards it really be ethically problematic? A look must be taken at the effects which could fundamentally ensue as a result of further changes in conventional terminology regarding the body and attitudes towards it. It is not possible to predict in detail the future appearance and functions of the body under the influence of tissue engineering developments. And yet it is conceivable that human beings — due to increasing opportunities to replace defective tissue and organs — could in time feel alienated from their natural origins. If the body were increasingly to become a product of artificial interventions, from time to time requiring repairs and upgrading, then the distinction from other devices and machines around it would in time become blurred. The features distinguishing a human being from a machine or an artifact would also become increasingly vague. This 'artifactualization' could lead not only to feelings of alienation from one's own origins but also to increasing disorientation.

The artifactualization of mankind — i.e. development from a 'natural' body to one he has artificially created himself — would not be a unique development *per se*, however. Throughout the course of history, man's entire world has always been subject to permanent reshaping into a cultural product he himself has influenced. Most of this world is no longer in its original natural state. The human world has gradually ceased to be viewed as a non-violable gift of nature. Most human beings nowadays cover up their bodies with textiles, for example, and surround themselves with man-made cultural products, like houses, cars, parks and towns. Against this background the increasing artifactualization associated with tissue engineering does not appear as a development which is either completely new or dramatic. It could rather more be perceived as the logical continuation of a long ongoing process of general artifactualization of nature, or as its mere extension to the human body. However, the feelings of alienation, disorientation and anxiety which this process could provoke do not just disappear as a result of these contemplations. In themselves they remain undesirable.

5.5 Conclusion

Evaluation of the research field objectives

The results of the analysis for the research field of tissue engineering first need to be viewed with regard to the two objectives behind it, namely to 'increase the therapeutic options available' and to achieve 'advances in research'. It may be concluded: both goals have an extrinsic value. The increase in therapeutic options which tissue engineering could maybe facilitate would contribute to the health and well-being of mankind. And the advances in research hoped for as a result of tissue engineering could positively affect the therapeutic possibilities. For researchers a possible increase in knowledge would also have an intrinsic value, holding the expansion of knowledge in high esteem *per se*. Both goals consequently appear desirable.

Contribution of the research field to realizing the objectives

The results of the analysis regarding the contribution of tissue engineering to actually realizing these two objectives reveal the following: In the light of progress made in the research field of tissue engineering to date, the development of new therapeutic options in the further course of research is certainly within the range of probability. The actual production of complete, complex organs is not yet possible, however. And whether it will ever become possible remains to be seen. The necessary know-how is simply not available yet. The great expectations held with regard to stem cell technology as the key to tissue engineering also remain unfulfilled to date. This research field still contains a number of significant scientific and technological problems, some of which may never be satisfactorily solved. Overall, however, it seems highly probable that the objective of increasing therapeutic options with the help of tissue engineering will be realized.

It also highly probable that the research field of tissue engineering will contribute to realizing the objective 'advances in research'. The extent to which individual advances in research will actually occur is of course unknown for now. It also remains to be seen whether and to what extent factually achieved advances in research will actually contribute to the development of new therapies.

Ethical problems

With regard to the ethical problems associated with tissue engineering, the analysis reveals the following: Potential problems of responsible development and appropriate use exist in conjunction with the issues of informed consent, data protection and the right (not) to know. According to the analysis, these problems are not fundamentally insurmountable. To recall just one example, the problem of data protection could be solved by destroying the data identifying the donor of a cell sample.

Problems intrinsically connected with the technology exist in conjunction with the type of starter cells used to produce replacement tissue and organs. The use of totipotent stem cells, for example, necessarily involves the ethically problematic destruction of embryos. From an ethical standpoint, use of this cell type is thus to be rejected. The use of pluripotent ES cells is also problematic — especially for supporters of the conceptionalist view. The acquisition of these cells inevitably involves the destruction and/or instrumentalization of embryos. By contrast, the harvesting of pluripotent EG cells — from the primordial germ cells of already dead fetuses — could, under certain circumstances, be ethically justifiable.

Problems linked to embryo protection could be totally avoided if only adult stem cells and fully differentiated cell types were to be used for the production of replacement tissue and organs. From an ethical point of view, research projects concerned with furthering the utilization of these kinds of starter cell are to be favored.

In the longer term two undesirable effects could result from tissue engineering. Firstly, if the theoretical possibilities currently envisaged for tissue engineering really were to be developed and then implemented, their enormous potential to realize various optimization wishes regarding the human constitution could provoke a growing feeling of discontentment, as well as lead to medicalization. In the course of practical developments in tissue engineering, human beings could come to regard various parts of their bodies — which they would currently consider to be functioning 'normally' — as 'below par' and therefore needy of treatment. It is also debatable whether, in the light of shortages in the health sector and the uneven distribution of means worldwide, medicine on request based on tissue engineering technology would be ethically justifiable at all.

Secondly, the changing attitudes of human beings towards their bodies in the course of further tissue engineering developments and applications could provoke feelings of alienation and disorientation, as well as anxiety about the future. These two negative effects are not necessarily inevitable, though. A discussion about possible ways of avoiding them would be both necessary and promising.

Ethical desirability

Overall, the first of the three conditions — which have to be met if the further development of tissue engineering is to be ethically desirable — can be deemed fulfilled with regard to the two objectives behind this research field, namely 'to increase the therapeutic options available' and to achieve 'advances in research'. The same is true regarding the second condition for both objectives. And the third condition can also be deemed fulfilled for both objectives.

Thus further development of the research field of tissue engineering is principally desirable from an ethical point of view with regard to both its objectives. Its further development can be pursued in a manner which is ethically justifiable. Whether this will actually *happen*, or whether in the future pursuit of this research field will deviate from the options shown to be ethically responsible in the analysis, remains open. The results can be summarized in the following overview:

Objective		Result regarding question no.:	Condition fulfilled:		Ethical desirability
Increasing the therapeutic options available	1	Objective really desirable	yes	1	
	2	Contribution highly probable	yes	2	principally yes
	3	Problems can be surmounted	yes	3	
Advances in research	1	Objective really desirable	yes	1	
	2	Contribution highly probable	yes	2	principally yes
	3	Problems can be surmounted	yes	3	

6 BIOELECTRONIC SYSTEMS

6.1 Research field

6.1.1 Bioelectronics

The field of bioelectronics is concerned with research into systems with a mixture of electronic and biological components (Willner & Wilner, 2001). This field has miniaturization in both information and communication technology in particular to thank for its recent progress.[1] This chapter will exclusively look at bioelectronic systems for human application, i.e. where humans or parts of humans represent one component within the bioelectronic system. In these applications electronic devices are often wholly or partly 'built in' to human beings. These bioelectronic systems integrate progress in prosthetic technology with progress in the computer sciences (Maguire & McGee, 1999). All other bioelectronic systems, which are not for human application, for example bioelectronic chips, are not investigated any further here.

The various bioelectronic systems for human application can be divided into two categories. The first includes systems where the electronic components interact *directly* with the human brain. Electrodes are fixed within the brain or to the head in order to receive certain impulses from or transfer impulses to the appropriate part of the brain. In the second category of systems the electronic component interacts *indirectly* with the brain. Electrodes are connected to functioning nerve strands which then pass on the signals transmitted by these electrodes to the brain.

6.1.2 Direct interaction with the brain

For a better overview of the bioelectronic systems which interact directly with the human brain, two different approaches can be dis-

---

[1] In the field of information technology, work began on large computing systems, progressing to desktops, then notebooks, then pocket-sized computers and recently to computers the size of wallets or even rings. In the field of communication technology, systems were first macrocellular, then microcellular, then wireless and now picocellular (Maguire & McGee, 1999).

tinguished: On the one hand, systems are being developed where special neuro-implants are fixed within the brain itself. A device located outside the body receives impulses which are then passed on to the appropriate part of the cerebral cortex via the neuro-implants. The brain is thus stimulated to process the signals. On the other hand, research is being done into systems where special electrodes fixed within the brain or to the head register electrical activity within the brain and then pass on this information to an electronic device outside the body. This device then converts the signals to various actions (Thomas, 1999).

Stimulation of the brain by an electronic device

The bioelectronic systems in this group include systems which convert certain visual stimuli from the environment to electronic signals and then use them to stimulate the visual cortex of the cerebral cortex. These nerve stimulation systems, also known as visual prostheses (Maynard, 2001), can be used in cases where blindness is caused by defects in the pathway to visual perception in the brain, yet where the neurons of the visual cortex are still functioning. This kind of blindness is quite common (Maynard, 2001). The systems can convert external light stimuli to electronic signals and provide a substitute for the stimulation of the visual cortex by the visual nerve which is no longer functioning (Brown, 1999; Maguire & McGee, 1999; Maynard, 2001). With the help of such visual prostheses, blind people could regain visual perception in the form of light spots, known as phosphenes, and thus be able to recognize faces, read texts or gain orientation in unknown surroundings (Maynard, 2001).

As far back as the 1960s and early 1970s, Brindley at the University of Cambridge (Brindley & Lewin, 1968) and Dobelle at the University of Utah (Dobelle & Mladejovsky, 1974; Dobelle et al. 1974) experimented with implants which they fixed to the surface of the visual cortex. Test persons were actually able to perceive phosphenes. Different experiments with blind people led them to believe that the visual system within the brain could possibly adapt itself to these unfamiliar visual stimuli (Normann, 1995; Normann et al. 1999; Dobelle, 2000). The blind people taking part in their experiments could see and read Braille dots faster, for example, than by touching them with their fingertips in the normal way (Normann, 1995; Thomas, 1999). The prostheses at that time, however, were not capable of creating several phosphenes which were close together and yet still clearly distinguishable. The perceptions were regularly sur-rounded by disturbing haloes, causing them to keep merging (May-nard, 2001).

Successes in the field of microelectronics have facilitated the devel-opment of microelectronic implants which no longer have to be fixed to the surface of the visual cortex, but which can actually be placed inside it (Normann et al. 1999; Maynard, 2001). Current research aims to develop implants with electrodes capable of stimulating only those few neurons in their direct vicinity. In this way, scientists hope to achieve a clear and differentiated visual perception — also of phosphenes right next to each other (Maynard, 2001). Another area of current research is animal experiments to investigate the risks of such implants, their long-term biocompatibility and the functional ability of visual prostheses implanted in the visual cortex (Normann et al. 1999; Maynard, 2001).

The visual prostheses currently being experimented on and which might become available in the future would principally be structured as follows: Firstly, they would have to contain a device — possibly a kind of video camera set into a special pair of glasses on the nose of the blind person — which would absorb external visual information. This device would convert the impulses to electrical signals and then pass them on to a computer-controlled electronic system — worn on the body or also integrated into the glasses. There they would then be converted to signals geared to the intracortical implant (Maynard, 2001; Maguire & McGee, 1999; Dobelle, 2000). These signals would then be transmitted to a three-dimensional implant set into the visual cortex and known as an *electrode array*, either via a special cable — for example subcutaneously near the ear — or telemetrically (Normann, 1995; Normann et al. 1996; Normann et al. 1999; Dobelle, 2000; May-nard, 2001). Each one of the many electrodes located on the implant set into the cortical tissue would then ideally stimulate a certain, restricted number of surrounding neurons (Normann, 1995; Nor-mann et al. 1999; Thomas, 1999; Maynard, 2001). In this way the blind person would receive a corresponding visual sensory impression which would probably at first be approximate to the pixel images on display boards in football stadiums (Dobelle, 2000).[2]

---

[2] Instead of to a camera, the system could possibly be connected to the television, a computer or the Internet (Dobelle, 2000).

A number of problems still have to be solved before visual prostheses could become viable in clinical practice, however. In addition
to issues such as the abovementioned biocompatibility and risks of
such implants — for example the risks of infection or rejection, or the
matter of how the cells in the visual cortex would react to permanent
electrical stimulus (Normann et al. 1996; Normann et al. 1999;
Dobelle, 2000; Maynard, 2001) — it is also necessary to achieve clarity regarding the issue of how exactly the brain interprets the stimulation pattern from the hundreds or even thousands of implanted
electrodes. It is not yet at all clear, for example, whether electrical
stimulation of the visual cortex in accordance with a particular pattern really does give rise to a correspondingly 'patterned' visual perception (Normann et al. 1999; Maynard, 2001). And how exactly
could electronic stimulation be used to achieve perception of different colors, textures or depths (Dobelle, 2000; Maynard, 2001)? Despite
all these open questions, scientists at work in this research field are
confident that in the future it will become possible to manufacture
visual prostheses suitable for clinical application (Normann, 1995;
Normann et al. 1999; Dobelle, 1998 & 2000; Maynard, 2001).

Stimulation of an electronic device by brain waves

This approach attempts to deduce from an electroencephalogram
(EEG) the characteristic patterns of electrical impulses in the brain
accompanying, for example, the raising of a finger, the speaking of a
word or the solving of a puzzle. The objective behind this research is
to use these patterns to control electronic devices. In this way
attempts are made to reinstate paralyzed patients with some of their
lost skills — for example to give back patients with amyotrophic lateral sclerosis[3] their ability to communicate. The idea behind this
approach is as follows: The database of a computer system would be
filled with different brain activity patterns, as well as their corresponding actions. From a patient's EEG the computer would then
decode the activity pattern corresponding to a particular action or
word thought of by the patient. It would compare it with previously
learned patterns and would then trigger the action or write the word
on a screen. Various bioelectronic systems are already being devel-

---

[3] Amyotrophic lateral sclerosis is a systemic disease of the spinal cord which
causes the nervous system to degenerate. In the course of the disease one of the
things patients lose is their ability to communicate.

oped on the basis of this approach — the utilization of characteristic activity patterns (Thomas, 1999).

A whole series of difficulties is involved in the realization of this approach, however. For example, an EEG is extremely difficult to analyze as it only returns the activity of the different neurons *en gros*. In addition, the patient in question has to learn how to control the activity of his brain consciously. In order to guide a light spot over the screen of his computer, for example, he first has to learn the 'thought' that goes with it (Thomas, 1999). The transmission rate of thoughts to a computer which 'records' them is also very slow. What can be achieved by learning to control one's own EEG signals lags far behind the potential of keyboard and mouse. This is due to the very narrow range of interfaces between the brain, with its multitude of nerve connections, and the computer, equipped to perform millions of computing operations (Thomas, 1999).

Another approach is the implanting of special devices in the motorial center of a patient's brain. Electrodes absorb the cerebral activity occurring there, and a minicomputer converts it into corresponding stimuli to control external devices — e.g. a cursor or a wheelchair (Maguire & McGee, 1999).

6.1.3 *Indirect interaction with the brain*

Bioelectronic systems in which the electronic component interacts indirectly with the human brain exist in the areas of *sensory replacement* and *motorial replacement*.

Sensory replacement

Bioelectronics researchers are already active in conjunction with all the human senses — (1) sight, (2) hearing, (3) taste, (4) smell and (5) touch — with varying degrees of success to date. The primary objective behind all this research is to help people who are wholly or partly lacking one or more of their senses to (re)gain their sensory perception. The technological approach chosen depends on the precise somatic defect causing the sense in question to fail. Causes can range from congenital defects to defects resulting from diseases or accidents to sensory failure in old age.

1) Sight

The rear part of the eyeball, which is normally hidden, is cased in three membranes. The outermost, protective case is the so-called sclera. Directly below this is the choroid. This in turn nourishes the innermost membrane, the retina. This last layer is light-sensitive. The retina contains millions of sensory cells, divided into rods and cones. These photoreceptors are stimulated by light entering the eye. Ganglia — the fibers of which form the optic nerve — then pass on the received stimuli as electrical signals to the visual center in the brain, where the image is formed which we see. The sensitivity of the retina varies in different areas. So-called rods make it possible to see at twilight and night; they cover most of the retina. So-called cones, on the other hand — facilitating focused image perception, as well as color perception — are chiefly located at the center of the retina, the so-called macula. Progressing from the macula to the edge of the retina, the proportion of rods increases and the proportion of cones decreases.

Sight may deteriorate when sensory cells in the retina die. This may be due to a disease, such as the hereditary disease *retinitis pigmentosa*. Or, as a result of the aging process, the macula may begin to degenerate. With these kinds of sight defect the ganglion cells located on the front of the retina are not affected. Scientists are exploiting this fact by attempting to develop bioelectronic systems to replace the failed functions of the retina. They hope to enable patients with defective sensory cells but with an otherwise intact visual system to see. Around the world various research teams are working on the development of implantable sight prostheses such as these. The two following approaches are to be found in the current research.

In the first approach a microcontact foil is inserted epiretinally (between the photoreceptors and the ganglion cells) in the damaged area of the retina (Larkin, 2000; Maynard, 2001; Wyatt, 1996). It is then connected to the functioning ganglion cells on the side of the retina facing the lens. The job of the implant is to make these cells pass on electrical signals to the visual cortex in the accustomed manner (Brown, 1999; Maguire & McGee, 1999).[4] The signals stem from a miniature camera or a microchip — located perhaps in a special pair of glasses on the nose of the patient (or in the future maybe in a contact lens). The camera receives visual information, converts it to electrical signals and transmits it wirelessly (e.g. using laser technology)

---

[4] For a detailed description of this approach, see http://www.uak.medizin.uni-tuebingen.de/subret/; site visited 1 August 2004 & http://rleweb.mit.edu/retina/; site visited 1 August 2004.

to the implanted contact foil (Brown, 1999). Scientists began to develop implants like this in the late 1980s. Since then they have been tested on patients. With their help patients could see a pattern which corresponded to the electrode simulation created on the part of their retina containing the contact foil (Brown, 1999).

In the second approach highly-sensitive microphotodiodes made of silicon, also known as a 'silicon retina', are implanted between the pigmented epithelium and the layer of photoreceptors. The retinal chip with its numerous photodiodes is thus implanted (subretinally) underneath the no longer functioning visual cells (Larkin, 2000; Maynard, 2001; Wyatt, 1996). Here the photodiodes — instead of the camera or the microchip in the first approach — convert light entering the eye into electrical impulses. Via electrodes connected to the tiny photodiodes, they then stimulate the still intact nerve cells of the retina to instill a visual perception in the brain once the signals have been passed on (Brown, 1999).

The visual bioelectronic systems presented here are not capable, however, of completely reinstating a patient's sight. Various essential questions must be clarified before clinical applications can be attempted in the blind or the severely visually impaired. Examples of the problems being addressed by current research are rejection reactions, long-term stability, permanent exposure of nerve cells to bioelectronic systems and toxic influences (Maynard, 2001; Normann et al. 1996).

2) Hearing

Good hearing depends, among other things, on well-functioning acoustic hair cells on the organ of Corti in the cochlea — the small snail-shaped duct in the inner ear. Sound is conducted through the outer ear via the middle ear into the inner ear. There the acoustic hair cells register the soundwaves, convert these mechanical signals to electrical impulses and then pass them on to the auditory nerve. The nerve impulse is preprocessed several times along the auditory pathway leading to the cerebrum — for example in the processing centers of the brain stem. In the auditive section of the cerebrum all the auditory information is ultimately pieced together to result in auditory perception.

If the hair cells in the inner ear are defective or completely destroyed — as a result of very loud noise, certain diseases or aging — insufficient or even no acoustic information can be absorbed and

passed on. The person in question is hard of hearing or deaf. And yet
in such cases the auditory nerve often remains intact. A conventional
hearing aid is of little to no help, providing merely an amplification
of the mechanical acoustic signals which such a person is barely
capable of receiving, if at all.

One answer can be special bioelectronic systems, known as
cochlear implants. To be successful they require the auditory nerve to
be intact. Surgeons implant a series of electrodes in the cochlea, at
exactly the point on the organ of Conti where the hair cells are defective or dead. There these electrodes receive electrical impulses from
an amplifier, known as a *speech processor*, which is carried extracorporeally like a Walkman.[5] The electrodes then transmit these
impulses directly to the auditory nerve. The speech processor has the
function of converting received mechanical acoustic signals into
coded electric signals and then passing these on to the electrodes
implanted in the cochlea. It receives the signals via a microphone
affixed in the proximity of the auricle. Via a special cable the coded
electrical signal arrives at a magnetic coil attached extracorporeally to
one of the temples. This coil passes the signal on to a second magnetic coil located under the scalp, which in turn is linked to the electrodes in the cochlea. Auditory perception results (Gezondheidsraad,
2001a).

As early as 1957 initial experiments took place to stimulate the
auditory nerve directly using electrodes (Djourno & Eyries, 1957). In
the 1960s and 1970s more systematic investigations were then performed in the United States, followed by the first successful implantations (House & Urban, 1973; Simmons, 1966; cf. House, 1995). The
single-channel system first used was less than satisfactory, however.
The breakthrough in cochlear implants came with the production of
multichannel systems (Gezondheidsraad, 2001a). In 1985 the American *Food and Drug Administration* (FDA) authorized the sale of two
cochlear implantation systems for use in adults with acquired
(postlingual) deafness. In 1989 the FDA authorized the use of
cochlear implants in children. By 2001 more than 40 000 people
worldwide had received an implant of this kind, approximately half
of them children (Gezondheidsraad, 2001a).

---

[5] As electronic systems become increasingly efficient, requiring less and less
energy, they can now be powered for a long time with very small batteries. As a
result, speech processors have been developed which are so small that they can be
worn behind the ear (Gezondheidsraad, 2001a).

The risks inherent in cochlear implantations are primarily linked to the surgical intervention involved, which can sometimes result in damage to the auditory nerve. The chances of this happening are very slight, however. This is also true of the postoperative risks, for example infection or wound necrosis. Long-term complications are almost unknown to date. The reliability level of the technique used for current implantations is very high. The lifespan of implants is estimated to be 15 years. The extracorporeal speech processor, with a current lifespan of 7 years, also appears to be technically very reliable (Gezondheidsraad, 2001a).

Technology relating to cochlear implants will very probably be developed further in future years. Desired future improvements include better sound awareness and a more precise adaptation of implants to individual patient requirements (Gezondheidsraad, 2001a). Further progress in the miniaturization of cochlear implant technology is also hoped for. This could maybe speed up the development of bioelectronic hearing systems located exclusively inside the body (Maniglia et al. 1999 & 2001).

In the course of progressing cochlear implant technology, different uses for it have been conceived. William House, for example, one of the pioneers in this research field, intended to use the new technology to enable the deaf to perceive surrounding noises (*environmental clues*) such as doorbells, voices, car noises, etc. Graeme Clark, the inventor of the multichannel system, wanted to help the deaf to do this and more, namely to understand speech. Other scientists have even aimed to integrate deaf people into the 'hearing society' (Reuzel, 2001).

We now know that the cochlear implant bioelectronic system does not provide a full substitute for normal hearing. And yet such systems can provide an important contribution to understanding speech, as well as to learning speech. For both sound awareness and speech comprehension, cochlear implants generally bring about a considerable improvement in the auditory perception of deaf children, provided that they receive sufficient post-implantation stimulation (Gezondheidsraad, 2001a). The utilization of cochlear implants also opens up possibilities regarding voice control. This technology can represent an important aid in the acquisition of speech for children who have been deaf since birth. It is now generally acknowledged as a method of treating children and adults who have lost their hearing (postlingual deafness) (Gezondheidsraad, 2001a; NIH, 1995). Many countries are still discussing the early implantation of such hearing replacement systems in the auricles of young children with congenital (prelingual) deafness (Gauntlett, 1996; House, 1986; see 6.2.2).

3) Smell

Our sense of smell can deteriorate with age, but also as a result of certain diseases. Two hundred thousand people per annum undergo medical treatment for olfactory and gustatory problems in America alone (Brown, 1999). With this in mind, bioelectronic systems which recreate a sense of smell could represent a potential form of therapy in the future. However, many aspects of the complex way in which the human sense of smell arises are still unknown (Schweizer-Berberich et al. 1995). This is one of the reasons why the so-called 'electronic noses' currently under research are very poor at mimicking the human sense of smell (Göpel et al. 1998).

An electronic nose is a device built from an array of sensors which is capable of recognizing various smells with the help of a pattern recognition system (Gardner & Bartlett, 1994). This device is not really a bioelectronic system in the true sense of the word, however, for it has yet to be integrated in a human organism. The electronic noses which are already commercially available are used in the classification and quality control of foodstuffs and coffee, beer, wine etc. (SA, 2001; Schweizer-Berberich et al. 1995).

There is a huge discrepancy between the way in which commercially available electronic noses function and the way in which the human nose functions. And at present it is unclear whether real bioelectronic systems which could recreate a lost sense of smell could ever be developed successfully. If it were to become possible, however, it would be conceivable that such systems could, if appropriately miniaturized, be placed within the nose. Potentially they could even go beyond mere recreation and expand upon human olfactory powers (Brown, 1999).

4) Taste

Usually the human sense of taste remains acceptable throughout a lifetime (Brown, 1999). The gustatory organ is linked to the human sense of smell, however. Any deterioration in the latter also has a negative effect on the sense of taste (Brown, 1999). Procedures like chemotherapy can also have a negative effect on gustatory ability. The first electronic tongue was developed in 1998. It was equipped with chemical sensors and intended to help in the detection and analysis of dangerous or disgusting substances like urine, blood or bad foodstuffs. Further potential applications for this electronic system were the testing of water for its potability or for the existence of viral bacteria. At the present time it remains unclear whether such systems could in the future be capable of manipulating the human sense of taste (Brown, 1999).[6]

5) Touch

Our sense of touch fulfills various tasks, for example the prevention of injury from hot or sharp objects. Without our sense of touch, we would get no feedback upon dropping something. And we would not know how hard we could grasp something without damaging it. Our sense of touch is thus an essential prerequisite for differentiated motor skills (Haugland & Sinkjær, 1999).

A first approach towards recreating touch is the development of a computer to replace the missing commands in the brain as reactions to certain signals from the tactile receptor cells — for example in the fingers. This computer would receive the signals passed on to the electrodes fixed around a nerve by the receptor cells in the fingers when they touched a certain object, and it would react accordingly, first relaying the optimum strength with which the hand should grasp this object, and then sending corresponding stimuli to the appropriate muscles (Haugland & Sinkjær, 1999). The objective behind this approach is the development of a bioelectronic system which, like the brain, can distinguish which of the many receptor cells in a certain part of the body is passing signals on to a nerve at any particular moment. In this way a patient could react far more sensitively to particular contact stimuli. This would, however, first mean the creation of electrodes which would be more sensitively connected to the nerve paths in question (Strauss, 1999).

A second approach to recreating the sense of touch, which is already being tested on patients, does not involve a computer deter-

---

[6] To date two 'antenna molecules', known as TR1 and TR2, have been discovered on the surface of the taste buds responsible for the perception of sweetness and bitterness. Researchers are still trying to find the two molecules relating to the perception of saltiness and sourness. In time, manipulation of the taste receptors could maybe facilitate the tasting of foodstuffs with a particular degree of sweetness or enable the bitterness of certain medication to cease to be perceived as negative (Brown, 1999).

mining the appropriate reactions to signals received from the receptor cells; instead, researchers are aiming to use intact 'feel zones' on the body to process incoming signals. Controlling whether a person who is paralyzed by a transverse lesion of the cord is standing upright and balanced, for example, functions as follows: Tactile electrodes on the feet of the patient send signals to his right and left shoulders. If the signals feel the same, the patient knows he is balanced. This approach is also being tested in patients who have lost total control of their limbs. Foot amputees, for example, can be fitted with a prosthesis which can send signals — calculated from the force with which the prosthesis contacts the ground — to an intact part of the body, e.g. the calf. The patient can then tell whether he needs to put his prosthesis down more firmly or not (Strauss, 1999).

A third approach, also currently being tested, involves connecting prostheses directly to severed nerve endings. However, in this case the nerve fibers coming from the spinal cord must be fully functioning. The electrodes protruding from such prostheses — e.g. a false hand — stimulate a special number of nerve fibers responsible for passing on a particular feeling to the brain — e.g. touching of the amputated thumb. These systems are already being tested on patients (Strauss, 1999). Ideally, such systems could replace all the feelings and capabilities of missing limbs (Strauss, 1999). In this case they would also be equipped with pain and temperature sensors for protective sensitivity.[7]

Motorial replacement

In cases where a patient has had an accident or disease which has destroyed only the nerve connections necessary for certain movements, in principle his corresponding muscles could still be functioning perfectly. Researchers are now using this fact in their search

---

[7] Our comprehension of the relationships between stimulus and perception is still minimal, however. It is therefore very difficult to mimic complex perception — e.g. not just the appropriate gripping of an object, but also perception of its texture. So far only replacement systems for individual perceptions have been successful. Research is now being done, for example, into so-called haptic devices for the perception of different tactile stimuli. If scientists managed to refine artificial touch to such an extent that tactile stimuli could be received from a remote location or a virtual reality, then this could also serve non-therapeutic purposes. For example it might be possible — dressed in a kind of diving suit — to have haptic interactions with a virtual environment in the form of 'cybersex' (Strauss, 1999).

for a method to replace seized-up motorial functions. The principle they are employing is as follows: movements which the patient can still perform are put to use. The shrugging of a shoulder, for example, can activate electrodes affixed there. The latter pass on the 'shrug' signals to a computer, which interprets them as corresponding commands and then passes these on to electrodes located elsewhere, for example the upper arm. They in turn transmit corresponding electrical signals of movement to, say, the muscles responsible for clenching the fist (Strauss, 1999). Ideally, a patient would thus be able to use selected intact body movements and an electronic prosthesis to trigger sophisticated motion. To date patients are able to move up to 10 muscles simultaneously using such bioelectronic systems.[8]

A second approach to recreating motoricity, which is still being tested, is as follows: In patients with amputated limbs, scientists are using the intact nerve strands between the stump and the brain to control prostheses. The nerves and muscles responsible for moving the amputated part of the body are directly connected to corresponding bioelectronic systems. In this way a patient whose hand has been amputated, for example, can operate a computer mouse or keyboard (Strauss, 1999).

6.2 Evaluation of the research field objectives

6.2.1 *Objectives*

Increasing the therapeutic options available

Bioelectronic systems research is aimed at increasing the therapeutic options for patients with sensory, motorial or cognitive defects (Kaku, 1997; Maguire & McGee, 1999). For many of these defects either no treatment exists to date, or the treatment available is less than satisfactory. For example, there is not an adequate therapy worldwide for visual impairments resulting from retinitis pigmentosa or degeneration of the macula. The latter is the most common reason why the elderly lose their sight. In the United States alone, 1.2

---

[8] Researchers are also developing systems based on changes in cerebral activity patterns. Patients would move their limbs by performing particular mental tasks (Strauss, 1999).

million people suffer from degeneration of the macula and approximately 10 million from retinitis pigmentosa (Kaku, 1997). Sensory, motorial or cognitive defects can have a significantly detrimental effect on quality of life.

The research field of bioelectronics is not aimed solely at using bio-electronic systems to alleviate the negative effects of such defects, however. Researchers are also trying to find ways of completely reinstating patients with lost motorial, sensory and even various cognitive abilities (Maguire & McGee, 1999). Methods are being developed, for example, to reinstate visual, communicative and motorial skills. Researchers are also trying to find ways of eliminating memory loss and progressive neurological diseases. Bioelectronic research is thus, to a certain extent, directed at the biomedical realization of recuperation from and treatment for defects which were previously only conceivable with the help of divine intervention (cf. e.g. Mark 8,22f; Matt 20,2; John 9,1f (healing of the blind); Mark 7,31 (healing of the deaf) or Mark 2,1f; Matt 9,1f; Luke 5,17f (healing of the lame)).

In the face of an ever-aging population — demographic trends are showing this development, at least for Europe — the therapeutic potential of bioelectronics as envisaged by the advocates of this research field has a particular significance. With age the probability of a sensory, motorial or cognitive defect increases, meaning that the overall number of such defects in the population will rise. The demand for bioelectronics will therefore grow.

Improving sensory, motorial and cognitive abilities

In addition to the development of bioelectronic systems to recreate lost abilities, the research field of bioelectronics is also aimed at finding ways of improving human abilities (Kaku, 1997; Kurzweil, 1999; Maguire & McGee, 1999; Mizrach, *year not given*). In all the three areas of (1) sensory, (2) motorial and (3) cognitive abilities, methods of improvement are being worked on. If these were to prove successful in the future, bioelectronic systems would also benefit healthy human beings.

1) Regarding the improvement of human *sensory* abilities using bioelectronic systems, there is current speculation about connecting up the natural eye to an artificial eye, for example. Ideally, the artificial eye would have better and more universal vision than the natural one. With such an eye human beings could maybe see wavelengths previously invisible to them — e.g. infrared — or things too far away

or too microscopically small for the natural eye to see (Kaku, 1997). Researchers are also pursuing ways of using bioelectronic systems to facilitate the perception of sounds which the natural ear cannot hear — because they are too high, too low or too quiet. Bioelectronic methods are being sought whereby the natural human olfactory organ could be empowered to detect smells previously far too faint. The possession of selected improved sensory abilities, made possible by a bioelectronic system — for example the ability to smell explosives or gunpowder and/or the possession of 'telescopic' vision — is an attractive proposition for members of certain professions. For a soldier, for example, having an implant at his disposal which could enable him to smell landmines could save his life (Maguire & McGee, 1999; Thomas, 1999). With the aid of a special bioelectronic system — such as a special pair of glasses and a filter system implanted in the brain — a police investigator could be capable of fixing certain images potentially useful to an investigation and then retrieving them later for a more thorough study. In this way an officer could 'record' the faces of anybody attempting to flee from a building being searched. Traffic officers could recognize the number-plates of cars speeding past them.

In addition, there is great speculation in the field of bioelectronics about the possibility of combining the sensory abilities of various individuals (Warwick, 2000). One idea is the simultaneous implantation in several people of bioelectronic systems facilitating particular sensory skills, and then to link up these systems. Maybe, depending on the type of link, individuals could in this way perceive not only their own images, noises, smells and/or tastes, but also the impressions received by the other linked individuals. Here too, it is easy to see why this possibility of 'extended' sensory perception would be attractive to certain professions — again the military or the police spring to mind. The linking of various sensory impressions could be useful when pursuing criminals, for example. In court cases a reconstruction and witnessing with one's own eyes of a course of events could greatly simplify a prosecution.

2) Regarding the improvement of human *motorial* abilities using bioelectronic systems, research is being done into 'supernaturally' fast running or 'supernatural' muscle power. Different professions would be interested in the development of such bioelectronic systems. With the help of such systems, soldiers could defend themselves better against attackers or flee faster. Nurses might be inter-

ested in the development of a bioelectronic 'suit' which would enable them to lift heavy patients without any difficulty (Hadfield & Marks, 2001). Other examples where certain professions could benefit from the development of bioelectronic systems to improve motorial function are easy to think of.

3) Regarding the improvement of human *cognitive* abilities using bioelectronic systems, it may become possible to develop ways of enhancing the memory — in the sense of being able to store and retrieve larger quantities of new information. In this way a new language could be learnt or a new area of work mastered at greater speed. Also conceivable would be invisible communication with persons in different locations — known as *cyberthink* (Maguire & McGee, 1999, Warwick, 2000). Cyberthink would be greatly beneficial in situations requiring quick decisions. In time conventional communication by telephone could even become superfluous. Cyberthink could maybe even facilitate the development of new social communities mentally linked through this bioelectronic system.

Moreover, a chip could be implanted in the brain which would function as a kind of reference book. Then whenever certain questions are pondered it would be activated — as an image superimposed on the normal visual image, but without rendering it invisible (Maguire & McGee, 1999). Somebody finding himself in unfamiliar surroundings, for example, could 'think up' a map showing his destination and directions to it.[9] Somebody having to express himself in a foreign language could retrieve the desired sentences from his 'inner screen'. And if somebody wanted to operate an unfamiliar device, the chip could provide him with the necessary instructions for each different button.[10] Another possibility could be in-built face recognition programs in the human brain. These programs could provide the name of — and maybe further information about — a person encountered.

---

[9] It is already possible to determine one's own location to within 10 meters using a satellite-controlled global positioning system (GPS).

[10] Steve Feiner, Blair MacIntyre and Dorée Seligmann, scientists at Columbia University, have already developed a system known as KARMA (*Knowledge-based Augmented Reality for Maintenance Assistance*). This system covers one of the user's eyes with a grid displaying, for example, instructions for how to use a laser printer. In order to determine its location, KARMA uses sensors affixed to objects in the physical world. The whole system is controlled from a desktop computer (see http://www.cs.columbiaedu/graphics/ projects/karma/karma.html; site visited 1 August 2004).

Once again, various professions could profit from such bioelec-tronic systems, this time to enhance cognitive abilities. For example, the military or the police would benefit from being able to commu-nicate with colleagues instantaneously in particular situations. Pro-fessional people regularly required to process large quantities of new information — e.g. scientists, politicians, attorneys or physicians — could also profit from bioelectronic systems able to link the human brain to diverse databases (Maguire & McGee, 1999). It would mean faster and more effective processing and storing of information, as well as permanent access to the information stored (Warwick, 2000). An emergency physician could retrieve the medical file of a seriously injured person (to find out about incompatibilities) within seconds, for example. Police agents could immediately compare the face of a suspect with the list of criminals filed. Even stockbrokers could ben-efit over colleagues without bioelectronic access, being able to react faster to changes in the stock market.

6.2.2 Evaluation

Increasing the therapeutic options available

Therapy, when understood as *restitutio ad integrum*, can be evaluated as fundamentally positive. If, in the long term, the research field of bioelectronics actually does contribute to restoring lost sensory, motorial and/or cognitive abilities, then this process will effect an alleviation of suffering and a restoration of health. As a means of realizing the desirable objectives 'health' and 'well-being', the increase in therapeutic options provided by bioelectronics could then be deemed extrinsically valuable.[11]

Despite this fundamentally positive evaluation, the following point should not be ignored: Not all patients want to be rid of their sound perception and/or speech comprehension 'defect'. Cochlear implant technology has met resistance in the deaf community, for example (Crommentuyn, 2000; Gezondheidsraad, 2001a; Reuzel, 2001). In par-ticular, two objections are repeatedly raised to the use of cochlear implants. Firstly, use of this technology would pose limitations on the 'culture of the deaf'. It would reduce the number of deaf people, which in time could mean the closure of various institutions for the deaf (Crommentuyn, 2000). Secondly, cochlear implant technology is

---

[11] See 5.2.2 for a definition of extrinsic values.

not yet far enough advanced. Relatively speaking, it would thus be better to be completely deaf and to feel totally accepted within a flourishing deaf community, than to attain semi-acceptable hearing and then have to exert oneself constantly within the newly accessible 'culture of the hearing' in order to even begin to be able to cope (Crommentuyn, 2000; Reuzel, 2001).

Throughout the development of cochlear implantation, debates have repeatedly taken place in the United States and in Europe about implants in children who are born deaf (prelingually deaf). These debates have been set in motion by various organizations for the deaf, as well as by parents of deaf children. In the 1990s protest marches were organized in many countries, including Canada, Denmark, Germany, Norway, Sweden and the USA, to demonstrate against the implantation of such systems in young children (Gezondheidsraad, 2001a). One of the standpoints put forward was that deaf people should no longer be viewed as 'non-hearing' and thus handicapped, but rather as members of a special community with its own culture and language (signing for deaf-mutes) (Gauntlett, 1996; cf. Reuzel, 2001). The advocates of this point of view saw cochlear implantation not as a helpful method in the treatment of deafness, but as a threat to the deaf community, or as an attempt to suppress its emancipation (Crouch, 1997). Various authors have countered this, however, with the reminder that most deaf children have hearing parents. In such cases, it is not a convincing argument to maintain that cochlear implants would pose a threat to the deaf community. Before having them, the hearing parents of these deaf children had no particular link to the deaf community. Consequently, they should be allowed to decide for themselves whether a cochlear implant would be advantageous for their child or not (Levy, 2002; Nunes, 2001).

Improving sensory, motorial and cognitive abilities

At first sight this objective seems positive. The very concept of improvement implies a positive evaluation. And yet a closer look reveals that it is not all that clear which changes in sensory, motorial and/or cognitive ability brought about by bioelectronics would actually be seen by an individual as being an improvement in the long term. Firstly, it could turn out that a particular improvement is only viewed as such in the short term. What seemed to be a positive change at the beginning could in time become the opposite. Secondly, the evaluation of changes brought about by bioelectronics is subjective. What for one person represents a positive change could for another be neutral, and for a third even be negative. The ability to see ultraviolet light, for example, could be viewed as a blessing or — as a result of the flood of additional impressions — as a pest. One person might be totally enthusiastic about being permanently connected to a database, finally able to quench his thirst for new information; for another, the permanent ability to call up the latest information could make him feel forced to do so at all times, leading to the excess of information becoming a burden. One person equipped with the bioelectronic communication system cyberthink might enjoy the permanent contact with others, whilst another person might after a while feel that his privacy has been infringed upon.

There is no real solution for the problem of estimating in advance which changes in sensory, motorial and/or cognitive ability would actually signify an improvement. Here there is no norm — of the *restitutio ad integrum* type for therapeutic interventions — determining which changes would constitute an improvement and which would not. On the other hand, one should not ignore the possibility that bioelectronic changes in sensory, motorial and/or cognitive ability could be effected which really would be experienced as a permanent improvement.

If for a moment we ignore the described difficulties surrounding advance estimation and just assume that human beings would be improved as a result of bioelectronic interventions, there is still the following problem to address: improvement knows no natural limits. Something which has already been improved once could then be improved again once technology has progressed further, and then again and again. The application of different bioelectronic systems to improve mankind would accordingly result in an ever more symbiotic connection between the human biological system on the one hand and the various technical systems at work on the other. This phenomenon is referred to as 'cyborgization' of the human body.

The expression *cyborg* is a combination of the terms *cybernetics*[12] and *organism*. Manfred Clynes and Nathan Kline first coined the word *cyborg* in an article about the prospects of space travel (Clynes & Kline, 1960; cf. Gray, 1995). They developed various strategies to

---

[12] The research field of cybernetics is concerned with the laws governing control processes, especially in technology.

optimize human survival in space. They believed it indicated that the human body should be adapted to suit the demands of space travel. In this way human beings could guarantee their survival in space. The required technological upgrading of the human body would be aided by growing knowledge about cybernetic processes. Biological evolution had already shown how physical functions could be extensively modified in order to adapt human beings to a radically altered environment. Now mankind should undertake similar modifications with the help of biochemical, physiological and electronic interventions in order to adapt itself to another new environment, i.e. space (Clynes & Kline, 1960).

The present conception of the cyborg as a mixture of human body and technology has its roots in Clynes and Kline's contemplations. The author likewise comprehends a cyborg as a system where technical and organic components are extensively and mutually integrated and cooperate with one another (cf. Haraway, 1991; Klugman, 2001). Cyborgization of the human body has been in progress for a long time now (Fink, 1999; Haraway, 1985). It began with the utilization of inorganic replacement body parts. Today, many physical functions can be manipulated, mimicked or replaced with the help of prostheses, corrective surgery or implants. The developments in bioelectronics will signify a far closer symbiosis of body and technology than has ever been the case to date, though (Warwick, 2000).

Two groups in particular, namely scientists and the military, have a special interest in the progress of cyborgization.[13] The *Media Lab* laboratory of the future[14] at the *Massachusetts Institute of Technology*, for example, is currently working on a research project dubbed 'wearable computing' (Mann, 1997). The objective behind this project is the development of information and communication technology which human beings can wear on their bodies. On the Media Lab website there are figures wearing non-transparent and semi-transparent visors in front of their eyes. Beside each visor there is a video

---

[13] The various aspects of human cyborgization are also a source of inspiration to many artists. See, for example, the Internet sites of Stelarc (http://stelarc.va.com.au/; site visited 1 August 2004), Horst Prehn (http://www.foro-artistico.de/english/program/system.htm; site visited 1 August 2004) and Keisuke Oki (http://synworld.t0.or.at/ level2/art/oki.htm; site visited 1 August 2004).

[14] In 1985 this laboratory was founded by Nicholas Negroponte, who was very successful at finding sponsors for his enterprise. Today, a large number of employees, scientists and auxiliary staff are researching the technologies of the future — with an annual budget of six figures.

camera and a small antenna. Around their bodies the figures wear cables held together with insulating tape, a processor unit on their hips and a whole series of batteries on their shoulders.[15] The website notes that further miniaturization would be required before this technology could be built into the human body. Computer systems and cerebral areas could then be directly linked. The website further states that it is fairly likely that this technology, which would facilitate a whole number of easily imaginable applications, will be developed very soon. Once the possibilities of bioelectronics have completely unfolded and the relevant systems have been integrated in the human body, the latter will have been transformed into a cyborg far superior to the body's natural version.

The military is the second large group interested in the progress of human cyborgization (Fink, 1999; Gray, 1989; Gray, 1993; Maguire & McGee, 1999). The United States military invests considerable sums sponsoring development of the 'future soldier', for example. The future soldier will possess an air-conditioned, total-body combat suit and will be networked with his colleagues. He will be linked to the information and communication network of his unit via a bioelectronic system located in his helmet, which will also contain video cameras providing him with information about his immediate surroundings. The soldier will have no direct contact with the outside world. Sensors will, however, enable him to perceive biological and chemical weapons or other poisons, as well as to register weather data. Finally, the soldier will probably be equipped with a so-called xenoskeleton — for jumping over very high obstacles, for example — and with additional extremities for operating complicated weapons (CNN, 2000).

The notion of human cyborgization has even triggered euphoric fantasies about a complete surmounting of human nature in a future post-human era. Supporters of this idea speculate about the possibility of overcoming death by implementing the processes taking place within the neuronal networks of the human brain in an electronic

---

[15] See http://www.media.mit.edu/wearables/; site visited 1 August 2004. The benefits of these *wearables* are still limited, however (Mann, 1997). In the Winter of 1994, for example, Steve Mann developed the so-called *Wearable Wireless Webcam*. This system transmits images from a camera fixed to the head of the user to a base station via amateur video frequencies. These images can then be followed on an Internet website, more or less in real-time. (See http://www.media.mit.edu/wearables/timeline.html#1994d; site visited 1 August 2004.)

medium (Kurzweil, 1999). In this way 'post-human man', totally fused with information technology, could continue to exist *in saecula saeculorum*. As an absolute cyborg, he would have totally liberated himself from his human nature and thus from all restrictions inherent in this human nature.[16]

Since no natural limitations exist in the area of enhancing bioelectronic interventions, human cyborgization — proceeding steadily with each new improvement — would also have no natural limitations. Yet unlimited cyborgization, pushed ever onward, could create serious existential difficulties for the individual. These difficulties would affect (1) his personal identity, and (2) his self-perception as a human being.

1) Personal identity

When a human being thinks about his own person, he particularly examines issues such as: What am I good at? How do I perform? Do I act responsibly? What is my particular character? What makes me unique? What can I remember? What is my life-history? If a human being were constantly subjected to new bioelectronic interventions to improve his sensory, motorial and/or cognitive abilities, it could become increasingly difficult to answer such questions. Improving the cognitive abilities of a human being, for example, could mean that his own mental efforts cease, becoming totally dependent on high-performance bioelectronic implants. As a result, that individual human being would find it increasingly difficult to say which results of his thoughts and actions still constitute a *personal* achievement. If not only cognitive, but also emotional improvement systems were to become available for implantation, it would become increasingly difficult to determine the characteristics specific to an individual. If, in addition, many different people were to share the possibility of being permanently connected to databases, the exclusiveness of possessing particular information would become relative, which in turn would reduce the uniqueness of those people.

Implantation of the cyberthink bioelectronic communication system — which would 'wire up' different individuals to enable them to exchange their conscious thoughts and experiences — could blur the

---

[16] In precise terms, a post-human, silicon-based creature would no longer be a cyborg, lacking its characteristic organic components.

borderline between the self and the cyberthink community (Dertouzos, 1997; Maguire & McGee, 1999).[17] In the face of such mental wiring, how are one's own thoughts and experiences and life-history to be kept separate from those of others? And the borders between the real world and the virtual world would become increasingly blurred. As a result, it would become more and more difficult with advancing cyborgization to determine one's own personal identity. In the long term this could even mean a dissolution of personal identity altogether. The mere thought of such a potential development causes human beings to become confused and disquieted. As a result, bioelectronic interventions to improve human sensory, motorial and/or cognitive ability cannot be evaluated as purely positive. A more detailed analysis of the effects of certain improving bioelectronic interventions on the person, his autonomy and his authenticity is definitely required, and yet a well-founded analysis of this type will only really be possible once clearer scenarios have crystallized. The future scenarios outlined at present are too vague for an exact conceptual description or appropriate evaluation.

2) Self-perception as a human being

If bioelectronics were actually to develop with as much success as its advocates hope, the symbiosis between man and technology would become increasingly narrower. The cyborgization of mankind would proceed rapidly. The process which this cyborgization would trigger, namely man becoming more and more a product of technology, can be referred to as human 'artifactualization'.

In recent times this process of artifactualization has been accompanied by a second process: technological systems are increasingly being developed along the lines of organic systems. This is happening in the fields of artificial intelligence, artificial life, robotics and neuronal networks, to name just a few examples. In the long term it is hoped that certain technological systems will be able to imitate various human or animal skills. After the artifactualization of human beings, this process can be termed an 'anthropomorphization' of technology.

The combination of these two processes, the artifactualization of human beings and the anthropomorphization of technology, could in

---

[17] Moreover, non-wired persons could find themselves under great pressure from the cyberthink community to become wired themselves (Klugman, 2001).

time lead to the following problem: pairs of opposites which have been around for hundreds of years, like 'nature — culture', 'organic material — inorganic matter', 'conscious subject — unconscious object', could become fuzzy. And yet for a very long time such pairs of opposites represented essential elements within human self-perception. A fuzziness would mean the necessity of fundamentally changing human self-perception to fit the new situation. In the face of the artifactualization of human beings and the anthropomorphization of technology, what exactly still belongs intrinsically to the 'nature' of human beings, to their 'humanity'? What is it about human beings that may not be violated if we do not want to run the risk of the 'typically human' disappearing? What exactly distinguishes human beings from artifacts?

Neither is it easy to answer the question of whether this increasing confusion regarding human self-perception has to be evaluated negatively. Here too, more detailed discussion and analysis are required, exceeding the framework of this book. It is possible to say at first sight, however, that even the thought of such developments gives rise to feelings of uneasiness, creeping disorientation and even existential panic. The very foundations of our image of mankind are shaken.

All in all then, the utilization of bioelectronic systems to improve human sensory, motorial and/or cognitive ability could mean fundamental changes in connection with human self-perception. Slow but sure cyborgization of a human being for his own improvement could have an effect on both his personal identity and his self-perception as a human being. The consequences these fundamental changes would have are very difficult to estimate in advance, however. This means that it is impossible to give a clear and conclusive evaluation of the objective analyzed here. The profundity of potential change does mean, however, that a detailed debate should commence in advance of developments.

6.3 Contribution of the research field to realizing the objectives

6.3.1 *Increasing the therapeutic options available*

In theory, therapeutic options for the treatment of sensory, motorial and cognitive defects could very possibly be increased. Few satisfactory therapies have been developed in these areas to date. In fact, many sensory, motorial and cognitive defects exist today which cannot be treated — either sufficiently or at all — using the non-bio-

electronic therapeutic means available. For example, people paralyzed by a transverse lesion of the cord cannot regain their motorial
skills. Also, blind people whose handicap stems from a defect in the
visual cells on the back of the retina cannot regain their sight with
existing therapies. These defects could possibly be eliminated with
the help of bioelectronic interventions. People paralyzed by a transverse lesion of the cord could — for example with the help of electronic prostheses — begin moving again. With a retina implant, blind
people could begin seeing again. The successful utilization of bioelectronic systems in these areas therefore would contribute to
increasing the therapeutic options available.

In a few sub-areas of bioelectronics, some modest results have
already been achieved in practice. And yet many therapeutic
approaches based on bioelectronics are still far from perfect. Often
they do not completely reinstate missing functions. Debate about the
present therapeutic value of cochlear implants is therefore not unreasonable (Reuzel, 2001). The visual bioelectronic systems in existence
so far do not bring sight back completely. It is not at all improbable,
however, that further progress will be made in the field of bioelectronics, and that therapeutic approaches will improve as a result. An
important role is played in this context by the miniaturization of
information and communication technology, a process which is generally expected to continue. And yet it is impossible to predict at the
moment the extent to which bioelectronic research will lead to real
and successful therapies in individual areas.

6.3.2 *Improving sensory, motorial and cognitive ability*

At first sight bioelectronic interventions in human beings are seemingly able to contribute to realizing this objective. On the other hand,
as has already been mentioned, guaranteeing any improvement in
sensory, motorial and/or cognitive ability as a result of these interventions is problematic. Bioelectronic modification might be seen by
one person as positive, by the next as neutral and by a third as negative. And certain, initially positive modifications might in time
become the opposite. There is no clear and fixed norm to character-
ize some modifications as improvements and others as non-improve-
ments. It is quite likely, however, that this problem might become less
acute as experience in this field grows.

Thus far, great improvements in sensory, motorial and/or cognitive ability may not be realizable with the help of existing bioelectronic systems. None of the improvements listed here is actually pos-

sible on the basis of current developments — with the exception of the experiment carried out by Kevin Warwick, Professor of Cybernetics at the University of Reading in the UK (Warwick, 2000)[18]. And yet various scientists are predicting that further progress in bioelectronics over the coming decades will facilitate sophisticated, enhancing bioelectronic systems (Maguire & McGee, 1999; Thomas, 1999). It remains to be seen just how true this will be for individual applications. The extent to which these enhancing systems would actually be practicable also remains to be seen, i.e. whether they could be satisfactorily integrated into everyday life.

6.4 Ethical problems

Ethical debate about the problems potentially surrounding further developments in the research field of bioelectronics has not really begun yet. There have already been debates about the use of cochlear implants (see 6.2.2), as well as about cyborgs — the latter incidentally currently colored by feminist, postmodern and anthropological standpoints (Haraway, 1985 & 1991; Gray et al. 1995). However, only a few publications have thus far appeared on real ethical problems connected with the research field of bioelectronics (e.g. Maguire & McGee, 1999; Mizrach, *year not given*).

6.4.1 *Problems of responsible development and appropriate use*

Risks

The risks to mankind associated with the new bioelectronic technologies are not easy to assess in advance (Maguire & McGee, 1999).

---

[18] In August 1998, Warwick had a silicon chip implanted in his arm. It was linked via radiowaves and a network of antennae to a special computer which could monitor Warwick throughout the Cybernetics Faculty building inside his University Institute. Via the network of antennae the computer was also able to react to various actions performed by Warwick. In the Institute entrance hall, for example, was a device which said 'hello' to Warwick every time he entered. The computer could follow Warwick's movements through the building, able to open the door to his laboratory and turn on the light for him. Warwick kept the implant inside his arm for nine days, during which period a simple movement of the arm could cause various things to happen. Warwick wanted to investigate with this experiment whether certain information can be received as well as transmitted by an implant. The experiment was successful, showing how the principles of cybernetics could be implemented in practice (Warwick, 2000).

On the one hand, they would be in the area of the surgical interventions themselves — the implantation, maintenance or upgrading of a bioelectronic system. On the other hand, they would result from the possibility that the human organism might not tolerate a particular implant (Maguire & McGee, 1999).[19] Since bioelectronic systems are still in the initial stages of their development and no sophisticated technology yet exists, it is difficult to estimate how these two risk areas will unfold in the future. The surgical interventions themselves could one day become absolutely standard interventions, for example, involving calculable and minimal risks. Materials could be developed which would not even harm the human body if implanted permanently.

In order to evaluate the acceptance of these risks potentially linked to bioelectronic interventions, a look will now be taken at their ratio to the concomitant benefits of the two bioelectronic categories — namely therapeutic and enhancing interventions. It is generally accepted that a certain proportionality should exist between the benefits of a medical intervention and its risks (Have et al. 1998). In addition, therapy is generally considered more beneficial and therefore fundamentally more valuable than enhancement. Enhancing interventions tend to be dismissed by society as unnecessary. After all, the body being enhanced is already healthy. To be consistent then, we may assume a greater readiness to accept risks associated with therapeutic interventions than those associated with enhancing interventions. We may also assume that society would be more likely, in keeping with the proportionality premise, to accept larger risks in connection with therapeutic bioelectronic interventions than in connection with enhancing bioelectronic interventions (Maguire & McGee, 1999).

There are, however, two things to be said about this. Firstly, we cannot rule out the possibility of the risks associated with therapeutic bioelectronic interventions becoming significantly reduced with growing experience. Since we can assume that any experience gained would also profit the category of enhancing interventions, the desired proportionality between benefits and risks could in time also be arrived at by this category. This would in turn raise the willingness to accept risks linked to this category. Secondly, it is impossible

---

[19] Incidentally, no significant problems have been ascertained so far in connection with human tolerance of cochlear implants (see 6.1.3).

to define clearly and unambiguously where exactly therapeutic interventions stop and enhancing interventions begin (Juengst, 1997 &
1998; Maguire & McGee, 1999; Parens, 1998). Just how bad would a
person's memory have to be before a memory-aiding bioelectronic
intervention could be categorized as 'therapeutic', for example? If the
intervention were to be performed 'too soon', it would be categorized
as 'enhancing'. As there is no exact distinction between bioelectronic
interventions 'geared towards therapy' and those 'directed at
enhancement', the risks associated with the different types of intervention cannot be clearly separated either. Overall, the issue of the
risks involved in the further development of bioelectronic systems is
unlikely to constitute an insurmountable ethical problem.

6.4.2 *Problems intrinsically linked with the technology*

Intervention in human nature

Another problem which sometimes rears its head in connection with
bioelectronic interventions concerns a potentially impermissible
intervention in human nature. The view often underlying this argument is that nature is morally good and technology morally bad (cf.
Maguire & McGee, 1999). This view can be interpreted in two ways:
(1) *All of technology* could be generalized as morally bad, with *all of
nature* being embraced as morally good.[20] (2) Only *bioelectronic technology* could be deemed morally bad, contrasting to *human nature* as
morally good. There are mighty objections to be raised to both of
these interpretations.

The following objection may be raised to the first interpretation:
Since his time on Earth began, man has always used different technologies to guarantee his own survival. One early example would be
the production and use of the hand-axe. The utilization of technology
can be viewed as inherent to human existence. Condemning all technology on principle would therefore amount to a radical condemnation of this elementary characteristic of human nature. And this
would appear to be counter-intuitive (cf. Maguire & McGee, 1999).
By the same token, it is not easy to defend a generalized positive
evaluation of all things natural. Considering all the different cruelties
of which nature is capable, deeming nature as totally free of moral

---

[20] Moral devaluation of technology often goes hand-in-hand with a fear of technology (cf. Achterhuis, 1998b).

blemishes poses problems and would not be in keeping with common sense. The first of the two interpretations is therefore extremely problematic.

There are also some objections to the second interpretation. Firstly, no reasons are given as to why exactly bioelectronic technology should be morally reprehensible. A categorical moral condemnation of a particular technology would be justified, for example, if more or less all the effects of that technology were to be negative, or if it could be comprehended as an exponent of a clearly immoral ideology. This would be the case with technology developed for torture purposes, for example. It can hardly be said to apply to bioelectronics, though. Research in this field is partly aimed at increasing the options for treating sensory, motorial and/or cognitive defects, after all. And various new therapeutic approaches have already been developed in this context. It therefore appears to be counter-intuitive to condemn bioelectronic technology as categorically immoral.

Generalized moral approval of human nature would only be justified if all human actions were either morally good or neutral. In the face of all the cruelties of which human beings are capable, however, its defense is riddled with problems. Generalized moral approval of human nature could be defended by maintaining that all cruel human acts are unnatural acts. But this would constitute an *ad hoc* hypothesis, based on an inadmissible *petitio principii*. Both interpretations are thus difficult to defend, rendering the problem of potentially unauthorized intervention in human nature — based on a morally dualistic evaluation of nature and technology — a pseudo-problem.

A variation of the 'unauthorized intervention in human nature' argument stresses the integrity of the same. Bioelectronic interventions violate the integrity of human nature, so the argument goes. This violation may be justified for some therapeutic interventions, but under no circumstances for bioelectronic interventions aimed at enhancement (Dertouzos, 1997).

Underlying this variation of the argument is the problem that there is no clear dividing line between bioelectronic interventions aimed at therapy and those geared towards enhancement. This view additionally lacks all explanation of why a breakdown in the integrity of human nature would be problematic only in conjunction with enhancing interventions and not with therapeutic ones. At first sight this even seems to be counter-intuitive. Some enhancing interventions in the integrity of nature *surrounding* mankind are even greeted with wide ethical acceptance, provided certain conditions are fulfilled. Why should human nature be so different? Overall, the 'unauthorized intervention in human nature' argument is difficult to support.

Playing God

Bioelectronic interventions could be interpreted as inadmissible interventions in divine creation. Accordingly, they would signify a wanton hubris towards God and thus an immoral interference in the divine order of things (cf. Dertouzos, 1997; Maguire & McGee, 1999).

This violation of a divine order argument provokes the following comment. First of all, it presupposes a theistic view of the world in which a Creator God plays the central role. This argument is thus only primarily valid for those people who subscribe to that premise. Let us suppose for the purposes of further analysis that a Creator God exists. Then we have to ask ourselves whether bioelectronic interventions really would interfere with the 'divine order of things'. In order to answer this we need to look at the Bible, first chapter of the Book of Genesis, verse 27. According to this text, God created man in his own image, in the 'image of God'. This verse can be interpreted in two ways: either God made man as a 'co-creator'[21], or God merely put man in charge of everything he had created in his own glory.

Taking the first interpretation, the playing God problem would then only be relevant if the following restrictions were imposed on the creativity fundamentally due to man: Either man is fundamentally prohibited from improving his sensory, motorial and cognitive abilities, this being an inadmissible intervention in Creation. Or man may improve his sensory, motorial and cognitive abilities, provided he does not do so with the help of *bioelectronic* interventions. The first restriction would lead, among other things, to the absurd consequence that the studying of any subject or the practicing of any sporting activity would already represent an intervention in the divine order and thus hubris. Besides, there is no theological justification for the special devaluation of *bioelectronic* technology in the second

---

[21] Pico della Mirandola was one of the advocates of this interpretation. He believed that God definitely instructed man to be creative in his own right (Mirandola, 1486).

restriction. It does not make any sense why God should be particularly opposed to this technology.

Taking the second interpretation of the Biblical verse, any attempt to improve upon Creation even in the slightest would be prohibited. All efforts of this kind would unequivocally amount to human hubris. To be consistent, man would only be allowed to preserve nature and not to change anything — neither negatively nor positively. And yet this view leads to absurd consequences. The desire for self-perfection inherent in man would be prohibited. Any fertilization of fallow soil, production of new foodstuffs, etc. would automatically mean human hubris.

Since the playing God argument does not stand up to the first interpretation of the Biblical verse, and since the second interpretation is so radical that it leads to absurd or at least indefensible consequences, upholding the playing God issue in connection with bioelectronic interventions appears to be problematic (cf. Maguire & McGee, 1999).

6.4.3 Undesirable effects in the longer term

Privacy and autonomy

A further potential problem is infringement of autonomy or privacy through the application of bioelectronic technology (Maguire & McGee, 1999; Mizrach, *year not given*). Standard use of bioelectronic interventions to improve cognitive ability in human beings would further intensify their links to computers. For example, contact to diverse databases would no longer be made via the fingers on a computer keyboard, but directly via the brain, which would be permanently connected to selected databases through an in-built bioelectronic information system. Standard use of enhancing bioelectronic interventions in human beings would also facilitate intensive links to other human beings. Communication with geographically remote people would then no longer only be possible via media like telephone or television, but also be permanently given — using the cyberthink communication system, for example — via a direct link from brain to brain.

Various side-effects are conceivable in conjunction with these applications which would facilitate easy access to the privacy of other human beings. The digital fragments left over every time a computer is used could help to retrace and register the exact movements and actions of a human being. The extreme networking of human brains would enable their visual impressions to be registered, their thoughts to be recorded, etc. At any one time a selected individual could thus be localized and registered in all respects — including his thoughts. Easy access to all areas of human privacy, even the most intimate, would then pave the way to subtle influencing and control. Direct networking of human brains would mean that human beings could receive — and subconsciously be influenced by — subliminal information. This would not only infringe upon the person's privacy, however, but also upon his autonomy.

One scenario which could gradually lead to an extreme violation of human autonomy in the long term may be painted as follows: Motivated by the enormous advantages to be gained from enhancing certain human abilities, the military could feel pressurized to keep up with the competition and equip its soldiers with the appropriate bioelectronic systems (Maguire & McGee, 1999). With sufficiently widespread military deployment of bioelectronic technology, an obvious next step would then be to develop a technology enabling the bioelectronic systems of the enemy to be controlled and influenced. In a society familiar with advanced bioelectronic technology, not only the military, but also the police and jails would be interested in systems able to control and influence. Such systems would, after all, enable wanted criminals to be traced and released criminals to be monitored. Corresponding systems could even be used to suppress undesirable human behavior. Maybe in this way criminal thoughts could be nipped in the bud. It would then be but a short step to the routine registration and control of citizens — to guarantee their own safety, but also to prevent supposedly disastrous situations. This would open the floodgates to direct influencing of the population in a direction desired by those in power. It is easy to imagine how keen dictatorial and absolutistic rulers would be to seize these opportunities to control and manipulate.

Social injustice

The further development and application of bioelectronic systems could in time lead to social injustice (Maguire & McGee, 1999; Mizrach, *year not given*). It is fair to say that modern society is very performance-oriented. Competition is rife in many areas of society. It is thus easy to imagine how society would be interested in bioelectronic interventions which could improve cognitive ability. These skills in particular are a decisive factor in the acquisition of a professional career, material wealth and social prestige. It is to be expected that parents would equip their children with bioelectronic systems to enhance their cognitive ability and then continually update them to outdo the competition and attain long-term success.

Generally speaking, social injustice arises as a result of social differences existing unfairly within a society. Nevertheless, social differences are not unfair *per se*. For example, it is often considered only fair that somebody who works harder and performs better should also earn more and be allowed to enjoy a higher standard of living. Unfair social differences only arise as a result of an ethically unjustifiable distribution of social goods such as status, prestige, money or employment.

Could the further development and application of bioelectronic systems bring about such an unjust distribution of goods? In order to answer this question, two hypothetical scenarios may be distinguished: In the first scenario bioelectronic interventions would be reserved for those who could afford to pay for them themselves; in the second scenario these interventions would be made available to everybody, without exception.

In the first scenario only the wealthy people in society would profit from the effects of enhancing bioelectronic interventions, i.e. only those who already enjoy a lofty social status and considerable material wealth. In this case, such interventions would cause the already unequal distribution of social goods to become more imbalanced. Those already privileged within society would continue to reinforce and improve upon their already outstanding social and professional positions. Additional opportunities for social and professional improvement would be made available to precisely those people already at the top of the social hierarchy. This can be deemed unjust. Firstly, it would further exacerbate the already unequal distribution of goods between the rich and the poor; and secondly, it would obstruct the principles within society of equal opportunity and solidarity with the weak.

In the second scenario, where bioelectronic interventions would be made available to the population at large, there would be no exacerbation of existing inequalities regarding the distribution of social goods. Anybody interested in doing so could undergo an intervention and profit accordingly. This scenario would therefore not promote social injustice.

However, bearing in mind the present shortage of money in the health sector, the first scenario — in which bioelectronic systems are reserved for the wealthy — would appear far more probable. Nobody is likely to take on board the enormous costs of a population-scale improvement in cognitive abilities.

Medicalization

Widespread bioelectronic interventions to enhance sensory, motorial and/or cognitive ability could be accompanied by the problem of medicalization (Maguire & McGee, 1999). It is quite probable that once a certain number of people have undergone enhancing interventions, others would feel themselves under increasing pressure to do likewise. Without such interventions they might fear not being able to keep up with those around them. In time, the attitude could become ingrained that in order to be successful in life one has to submit one's body to all the enhancing interventions available. As a result, attitudes towards conventional human abilities could change quite negatively in the long term. Average abilities could become almost akin to defects, in need of elimination. People could become afraid that their sensory, motorial and/or cognitive constitution is fundamentally inadequate. As a result, bioelectronic interventions could trigger a medicalization of thus far absolutely ordinary and normally functioning human abilities.

6.5 Conclusion

Evaluation of the research field objectives

The two objectives behind the research field discussed here are increasing the therapeutic options available and improving sensory, motorial and/or cognitive ability. The analysis reveals that the first objective has an extrinsic value. The increase in therapeutic options which bioelectronics could possibly bring about would contribute to the health and well-being of mankind. The first objective — leaving aside special cases where people do not wish to have their defects eliminated — therefore really does appear to be desirable.

Regarding the second objective, it would be good to be skeptical, however. Improving sensory, motorial and/or cognitive ability only seems to be unquestionably desirable at first sight. Taking a closer look, various issues appear problematic. For example, the effects of certain changes to sensory, motorial and/or cognitive ability might in time appear less desirable than originally assumed, or even negative. In the course of human cyborgization, a process driven along by bio-electronics, man would be in danger of encountering grave existential difficulties regarding both his own identity and his self-perception as a human being. These problematic issues prevent this second objective from being evaluated as clearly positive. Improving sensory, motorial and/or cognitive ability is not incontestably desirable.

Contribution of the research field to realizing the objectives

The results of the analysis with regard to the contribution of bioelectronics to realizing the two objectives are as follows. Regarding the contribution of the research field to the objective 'increasing the therapeutic options available', the verdict is positive. Further development of bioelectronics would very probably open up new ways of treating all manner of sensory, motorial and cognitive defects for which to date no other therapeutic means exist. The currently existing bioelectronic systems — e.g. the various systems for restoring sight or hearing — are only able to eliminate the defect in question in part, however, and cannot completely restore the lost physical function. It remains to be seen whether in the long term a complete elimination of sensory, motorial and/or cognitive defects could be achieved with the help of bioelectronics. Overall, though, further development of the research field would very probably contribute to realizing the first objective.

Regarding the contribution of bioelectronics to realizing the objective 'improving human sensory, motorial and cognitive abilities', it is harder to reach a positive verdict. At the current time, significant improvements have yet to be made to selected abilities with the help of available bioelectronic systems. Various authors predict, however, that further progress in bioelectronics over the next few decades will produce sophisticated enhancing bioelectronic systems. It remains to be seen whether this will be the individual case, however. It is also unclear just how practicable such enhancing systems would be.

Ethical problems

Regarding the ethical justifiability of the various problems associated with bioelectronics, the analysis reveals the following results. Problems of responsible development and appropriate use could arise in conjunction with the risks potentially involved in the application of new bioelectronic technologies, namely in connection with the required surgical interventions and with the tolerance of the body towards implanted bioelectronic systems. The actual extent of these risks cannot yet be estimated, however, since the development of different bioelectronic systems is still at the early stages. It is possible that the risks could be significantly reduced as empirical knowledge grows. In this analysis, the risks involved therefore appear to be an ethical problem which could potentially be surmounted. The problems intrinsically linked to bioelectronic technology comprise inadmissible intervention in human nature and the playing of God. Both of these were exposed in the analysis as pseudo-problems. To conclude, three undesirable effects could surface in connection with the further development and application of bioelectronic technology in the long term. Firstly, human privacy and human autonomy could be violated — especially in conjunction with bioelectronic interventions clearly aimed at improving certain cognitive abilities. These interventions would eventually pave the way to extensive control over other human beings. In addition, the application of 'enhancing' bioelectronics would be in danger of promoting social injustice. It is conceivable — and even very probable — that only the wealthy within society would be able to afford the enhancing interventions. Finally, the further development and application of improving bioelectronics could fan the flames of medicalization. In the course of its further development human beings could begin to regard certain aspects of themselves as requiring treatment which at the moment they consider 'normal'.

Taken overall, the ethical problems which could be involved in increasing the therapeutic options available therefore appear to be potentially surmountable and thus ethically justifiable. Regarding the objective of improving sensory, motorial and cognitive abilities, the ethical justifiability is questionable, however.

Ethical desirability

The overall results of the analysis regarding the research field of bioelectronics are as follows. Of the three conditions which have to be met, the first is fulfilled regarding the first objective — increasing the therapeutic options available. Regarding the second objective — improving sensory, motorial and cognitive abilities — its fulfillment is problematic. The second condition is fulfilled for the first objective. Regarding the second objective its fulfillment is likewise problematic. And the same is true for the third condition: it appears to be fulfilled for the first objective but its fulfillment regarding the second objective is problematic.

The further development of bioelectronics therefore appears to be principally ethically desirable with regard to increasing the therapeutic options available, following the criteria underlying this analysis. Regarding the improvement of sensory, motorial and cognitive abilities, on the other hand, its ethical desirability is questionable.

The results can be summarized in the following overview:

Objective		Result regarding question no.:	Condition fulfilled:		Ethical desirability
Increasing the therapeutic options available	1	Objective really desirable	yes	1	principally yes
	2	Contribution highly probable	yes	2	
	3	Problems can be surmounted	yes	3	
Improving sensory, motorial and cognitive abilities	1	Objective not clearly desirable	problematic	1	Questionable
	2	Contribution uncertain	problematic	2	
	3	Surmounting of problems uncertain	problematic	3	

7 GERM LINE GENOME MODIFICATIONS

7.1 Research field

7.1.1 *Germ line genome modifications*

A germ line genome modification is a change in the genetic material of a germ line cell (cf. Resnik & Langer, 2001). The human germ line is the cell sequence which unfolds during embryonic development, starting with the fertilized egg cell (zygote) and leading, without interruption, to the primordial germ cell of the embryo and then on to the germ cells of the sexually mature organism (gametes). Germ line genome modifications are either performed at the beginning of the germ line, on a fertilized egg cell or early embryo, or they are performed on the germ cells at the end of the germ line. The nucleus of a cell contains most of the genetic material of that person (nDNA). A small proportion is also located in the mitochondria, however (mtDNA).[1] As a result, germ line genome modifications can be performed on the DNA of the cell nucleus and on mitochondrial DNA. A change to the combination of nDNA and mtDNA in a germ line cell also represents a germ line genome modification.[2] Germ line genome modifications are usually inherited by offspring.[3]

---

[1] The main task of the mitochondria is to supply energy to the cell. Mitochondrial disturbances can lead to various diseases (Gezondheidsraad, 2001b; Lightowlers et al. 1997).

[2] One example of a germ line genome modification by altering the combination of mtDNA and nDNA is the IVONT-Protocol (cf. Bonnicksen, 1998a & 1998b; Gezondheidsraad, 2001; Resnik & Langer, 2001; see 7.1.5). A second example is the transplantation of the cell nucleus of a somatic cell to a denucleated egg cell (cf. Resnik & Langer, 2001; Schramm, 1999). A final example is ooplasm transplantation to treat a special kind of infertility (cf. Bonnicksen, 1998a; Gezondheidsraad, 2001; Resnik & Langer, 2001). In certain cases infertility in a woman can be caused by defective mitochondria. By introducing ooplasm from the egg cell of a donor, normally functioning mitochondria enter the egg cell of the patient to be fertilized (see 7.1.4).

[3] If, however, a genetic modification were to be performed on the mtDNA of a sperm cell, this modification would not be passed on to children. The mtDNA in the mitochondria is only passed on down the maternal line (Gezondheidsraad, 2001b; Lightowlers et al. 1997; Richter & Schmidt, 1999).

Germ line genome modification should be distinguished from so-called 'somatic gene therapy'. In the latter, it is not the genetic material of germ line cells which is modified, but that of somatic cells. In this group of gene-technological interventions, no DNA modification takes place within human germ line cells, meaning as a logical consequence that, in principle, no genetic modifications can be passed on to children.[4]

To facilitate a constructive ethical debate about gene technology in human beings, the bioethicist LeRoy Walters introduced a more precise distinction between the various gene-technological interventions in the 1990s. He categorized them not only according to the type of target cells addressed by the treatment — somatic or germ line cells — but also according to the aim behind the intervention — the prevention or therapy of disease, or the improvement (enhancement) of certain features. Using these criteria, he produced four categories for gene technological intervention in the human genome: 1) Therapeutic or preventive somatic interventions, 2) therapeutic or preventive germ line interventions, 3) enhancing somatic interventions and 4) enhancing germ line interventions (Walters, 1991). Walters' categorization had an enormous influence on the ethical debate at that time.

In 1995 the first ever protocol of an intervention in the human germ line was published (Rubenstein et al. 1995). This protocol — known as the IVONT protocol (*in vitro ovum nuclear transplantation*) — describes in nine steps the course of a cell nucleus transplantation from a female patient to a denucleated donor egg cell. The underlying goal was to replace all the mitochondria of the patient with those of the donor of the denucleated egg cell in order to prevent a mitochondrial genetic disease (see 7.1.5). This protocol was one of the motivations to add to Walters' four categories of gene technological intervention the further distinction of the genetic material type to be modified — the DNA of the cell nucleus (nDNA) or that of the mitochondria (mtDNA). Since then, a strict division has also been made between gene-technological interventions aimed at therapy and those aimed at prevention (Bacchetta & Richter, 1996; Richter & Bacchetta, 1998; Richter & Schmidt, 1999).

Criticism was also voiced regarding terms used regularly until then: somatic gene 'therapy' and germ line gene 'therapy'. With

---

[4] This is possible, however, if during somatic gene therapy genetic modifications are unintentionally made to germ cells (Resnik et al. 1999).

regard to gene-technological interventions in somatic cells, for example, the precise extent of their therapeutic potential is not yet clearly proven (Graumann, 2000). This technology is still at the experimental stage.[5]

With regard to gene-technological interventions in germ line cells, the regularly used term 'germ line gene therapy' implies the existence of an identifiable and sick person who is to be healed with the help of this kind of therapy. And yet at the time of the gene technological intervention there is no such person. It is therefore not strictly correct to speak of therapy in connection with gene-technological interventions in germ line cells, only really prevention or enhancement (Richter & Schmidt, 1999).

Finally, in the light of the wide range of currently researched possibilities surrounding the execution of genetic interventions — including the alteration of individual nucleotides of the nDNA or mtDNA, or the adding of artificial chromosomes to a germ cell (see 7.1.5) — the term 'gene' in the expression 'gene therapy' no longer seems appropriate either (Resnik & Langer, 2001).

For the abovementioned reasons, the author therefore deploys the expression 'germ line genome modifications' to refer to interventions in the genome of the germ line. This expression leaves room for both the precise goal underlying the intervention and for the actual genetic structures used — whether they be genes, nucleotides or whole chromosomes. And it also covers modifications to the nDNA of a cell nucleus, to the mtDNA of the mitochondria or to a combination of both (Resnik & Langer, 2001).

The technologies used to date for germ line genome modifications all originate from the research embedded in established science. Scientists can therefore be expected to continue making discoveries which could facilitate a further development of these technologies, regardless of whether they have germ line genome modifications actively in mind at the time or not. Four established research fields — each with its own development dynamics — will foreseeably play a role in the further development of germ line modification technologies: somatic gene therapy, fertility research, genetics and animal research (Stock & Campbell, 2000). The first of these fields is somatic

[5] The term 'gene therapy' became established in the literature as far back as the 1970s (Richter & Schmidt, 1999). Expressions coined without the term 'therapy', e.g. genetic surgery (Muller, 1965; Peterson, 2001) or molecular surgery (Temple, 1990) were, by contrast, not generally accepted.

gene therapy, currently receiving considerable financial backing. Various findings from this research field could be transferred to the field of germ line genome modifications (Stock & Campbell, 2000).[6]

The second field is fertility research (cf. Capecchi, 2000; Silver, 2000a & b). The *in vitro* fertilization technique (IVF) stemming from this field has developed over the past two decades to become an advanced method of reproduction for numerous couples otherwise unable to conceive (Stock & Campbell, 2000). The ooplasm transplantation technique developed within this research field already represents a kind of germ line genome modification (see 7.1.4).

The third research field mentioned above, genetics, will also have a significant influence on the development of germ line genome modification technologies (cf. Schroeder-Kurth, 2000; 2000a & b). It can be expected, for example, that discovery of the details of the human genome, as well as its functions, will create a basis for future genetic interventions and provide interesting opportunities for modifications to the genome of the germ line (Stock & Campbell, 2000).

Within the last field, animal research, applied molecular genetics and reproductive biology are being driven on worldwide by both academic institutions and private enterprises. The various aims behind this drive include the manufacture of low-price medication and the development of new types of cattle. Different findings from this research will probably play a role in the technologies used for germ line genome modifications in human beings, for example cell nuclear transplantation or the development of artificial chromosomes (Stock & Campbell, 2000).

7.1.2 *Germ line genome modifications in animals*

In the 1980s, first attempts at germ line genome modifications were made in various mammals — including mice, sheep, goats, pigs and cows (Frankel & Chapman, 2000). The animals emerging from these modifications are called 'transgenic animals' and are used, for example, as models for researching certain human diseases. With the help of various techniques, defective human genes are introduced to a particular type of animal in order to facilitate observation of the disease-producing effects of these genes, as well as the testing of various possible treatments. Different species of animal are also used in

---

[6] The technical challenges facing these two genetic interventions differ considerably, however (Capecchi, 2000; Resnik et al. 1999).

the production of selected elementary biochemical substances for human beings. Human proteins can be acquired from the milk of transgenic sheep, goats or cows, for example.

The generation of a transgenic mammal can be outlined as follows: Firstly, a suitable genetic construction, called a 'transgene', is developed. In simplified terms, this is done by bringing together a structural gene — coding the production of a particular human protein, for example — and a so-called regulator, an element to control the activity of the new gene in the recipient animal. Then the transgene is transferred to the germ line cells of the selected animal. This represents an attempt to integrate the genetic construction into all the cells of the future animal, including its germ line cells.

Various methods now exist for the installation of transgenes in the genetic material of animals. The first method described is also the one used most frequently. First, a number of egg cells from a mammal are fertilized *in vitro*. The genetic constructions are then transferred to the emerging zygotes (Frankel & Chapman, 2000) before the nuclei of the sperm cells have fused with those of the egg cells. This is performed using a micro-injection into one of the two pronuclei in each case (Seehaus, 2000). This procedure is very complicated and not particularly efficient. Only a low percentage of genetic constructions can be successfully integrated into the genomes of the offspring of genetically modified models. In addition, the genetic environment new to the foreign gene can have a negative effect on its expression.

A second method works with vectors suited to performing particular genetic modifications in embryonic stem cells (ES cells) (Resnik et al. 1999; Seehaus, 2000). Genetically modified ES cells are injected into embryos at the blastocyst stage. This leads to the development of so-called chimeras, i.e. individuals containing different genetic cells. Selected mating can then lead to offspring containing the new genetic construction throughout their cells.

A third method is transplantation of the cell nucleus of a somatic cell into a denucleated egg cell. This leads to an alteration in the original combination of mtDNA and nDNA. This technique has been used to perform germ line genome modifications in mammals — including mice, rabbits and cows. One of the most famous examples of its application was the creation of the sheep 'Dolly'. Scientists have already succeeded in cloning various types of mammal using reproductive cloning techniques. Nuclear transplantation of post-embryonic cell nuclei has facilitated the cloning of sheep (Wilmut et al.

1997), cows (Kato et al. 1998), goats (Baguisi et al. 1999), pigs (Pole-jaeva et al. 2000) and mice (Wakayama et al. 1998). Rhesus monkeys could only be successfully cloned, however, by transplanting the nuclei of preimplantation embryos (Meng et al. 1997; Wolf et al. 1999). Cloning experiments are currently being performed on hares, rats, cats, dogs and horses (PHC, 2002). The success rate for repro-ductive cloning in animals varies considerably, depending on the type of animal (Hill, 2002; PHC, 2002). Generally speaking it is low, both in relation to the overall number of embryos created in the lab-oratory using cell nuclear transplantation and in relation to the num-ber of embryos which have been implanted in the uterus to date (Byrne & Gurdon, 2002; Berardino, 2002; Healy et al. 2002; Hill, 2002; Jaenisch & Wilmut, 2001; PHC, 2002).

Problems regularly occur in connection with reproductive cloning in animals, starting during the gestational period. The number of spontaneous abortions, for example, is significantly higher in animals which have undergone reproductive cloning than in those which have undergone IVF treatment. Unlike with conventional pregnancies — where most fetal losses occur during the first third — the losses which occur following reproductive cloning are spread throughout the ges-tational period and into the early neonatal period. In addition, many anomalies can be observed in pregnancies resulting from cloning, for example abnormal development of the placenta, gestational toxicosis or uncontrolled fluid retention in the uterus (Hill, 2002; Jaenisch & Wilmut, 2001; PHC, 2002). A whole range of anomalies and defects can be observed in the tissue and organs of cloned animals once they are born. Animal clones are often born abnormally large or have prob-lems with their lungs, kidneys, livers, joints, immune systems, car-diovascular systems or brains (Jaenisch & Wilmut, 2001; PHC, 2002). The mother animals used for reproductive cloning purposes are also subjected to various health risks. Many of the problems connected with gestation following reproductive cloning — for example an abnormally large fetus or a spontaneous abortion — do not only amount to an increased risk to the mother's health, but sometimes even to a risk of her dying (Berardino, 2002; PHC, 2002).

7.1.3 *Somatic gene therapy in human beings*

The objective behind somatic gene therapy is to produce a therapeu-tic or preventive effect in the carrier of an unfavorable genetic struc-ture. This is attempted by transferring suitable genetic material to certain somatic cells of that carrier. Since 1989 clinical experiments have regularly been performed in this field (Graumann, 2000). More 1000 clinical trials addressing human somatic gene therapy are currently planned, already in progress or have been completed worldwide (GTCT, 2001).

The concept of using somatic gene therapy to cure or prevent certain diseases was initially greeted with widespread enthusiasm from both the scientific community and the public. Time has shown, however, that practical realization of the overwhelming theoretical possibilities is far more difficult than originally presumed. For example, transferring the new genes to precisely the tissue envisaged and then encouraging them to develop the desired expression there has proved problematic (Frankel & Chapman, 2000; Marshall, 1999). Basically, many of the hopes raised by somatic gene therapy are still waiting to be fulfilled (Resnik & Langer, 2001). First therapeutic successes have been achieved, however, for example in connection with the treatment of hemophilia B (Kay et al. 2000), as well as the immune deficiency disease SCID (Severe Combined Immuno Deficiency) (Cavazzana-Calvo et al. 2000).

The initial public euphoria regarding this new method of therapy and prevention was particularly dampened by the following occurrence: In September 1999 a young man named Jesse Gelsinger died in America following a somatic gene therapy experiment (Graumann, 2000; Marshall, 1999 Nordgren, 2001). An unexpectedly strong immune reaction to genetically modified adeno-viruses — transferred to Gelsinger's liver — played a role in his death (Graumann, 2000; Marshall, 1999). This event opened the eyes of the public to the various risks involved in the development of somatic gene therapy.

The media began by referring to Gelsinger's death as the first tragic loss in connection with the development of somatic gene therapy. Soon afterwards, however, they uncovered further deaths which had occurred previously to this one. They also discovered that various researchers and institutions in America had not reported negative findings from their somatic gene therapy research to the American health authorities, despite a previous agreement to this effect. As a consequence of these discoveries, some aspects of the regulations and methodology of clinical research into somatic gene therapy were subjected to a reevaluation (Barbour, 2000; Graumann, 2000; Nordgren, 2001). Furthermore, disappointment with somatic gene therapy increased after observing the development of a leukaemia-like disease as a result of gene therapy treatment with an adeno-associated viral vector for severe combined immunodeficiency (SCID) in two young French girls in 2002 and 2003 (Check, 2002 & 2003; Marshall, 2003). As a result of the tremendous impact of these adverse events, somatic gene therapy is seen as a hazardous procedure by both the scientific community as well as the public.

Two different approaches to the development of somatic gene therapy techniques are theoretically conceivable. In the first, the unwanted gene is left inside the genome of its carrier (Resnik et al. 1999; cf. Graumann, 2000; Paslack, 1999) and has the intact version of the gene added to it. The intact gene can be introduced in various ways. One method would be to transfer the new, intact gene to a chromosome of the carrier of the genetic defect. Various transportation systems have been developed to this effect, enabling the gene to be integrated within the chromosome. Another method would be to transfer the new gene to the DNA of a plasmid — a DNA strand, usually circular — which is then in turn transferred extrachromosomally to the recipient cell. The mechanism enabling this first approach to be realized is known as 'non-homologous recombination' (Resnik et al. 1999).[7]

In the second approach, the unwanted gene does not remain in the genome of its carrier (Resnik et al. 1999; cf. Graumann, 2000; Paslack, 1999). Instead, it is replaced by a new, intact gene. The latter is introduced to precisely the place in the chromosome of the carrier of the genetic defect where the defective gene was previously located. The mechanism in action here is called 'homologous recombination' (Graumann, 2000; Paslack, 1999; Resnik et al. 1999).

De facto only the first approach has been used in somatic gene therapy to date (Graumann, 2000; Resnik et al. 1999). The second approach has worked in human somatic cells (Russel & Hirata, 1998), but the success rate so far has remained extremely low. Scientists do expect it to improve, however, meaning that this approach might also be used in the future (Resnik et al. 1999). This would be desirable for the following reason: A new gene introduced to precisely the same genetic location as occupied by a previously removed defective gene would very probably become firmly integrated within the recipient

---

[7] A further approach in which the defective gene also remains in the genome of the carrier is the so-called 'blockade strategy'. Here an attempt is made to block the unwanted activity of a certain gene by introducing suitable genetic material (Graumann, 2000; Paslack, 1999).

genome. It would probably function normally and not alter the functions of other genes within the recipient genome (Capecchi, 2000). This would mean an elimination of the genetic defect. A gene added to the recipient genome using the method of non-homologous recombination, by contrast, might only have a temporally limited effect on cellular function. This would particularly be the case following introduction via an extrachromosomal plasmid. The result could be an insufficient correction of the genetic defect. There would also be a strong likelihood of the additional gene negatively influencing the functions of other genes within the recipient genome and thus damaging cellular function (Resnik et al. 1999).

7.1.4 Germ line genome modifications performed in human beings to date

Germ line genome modifications as a side-effect of somatic gene therapy

Somatic gene therapy is exclusively geared to modifying genetic material in somatic cells. During such interventions it can happen, however, that the genome of a germ line cell is unintentionally modified, too (Billings et al. 1999; Frankel & Chapman, 2000; Nordgren, 2001). The risk of this happening is very low (Gordon, 1998; Senior, 1999), but it cannot be ruled out completely.[8] The autopsy of Jesse Gelsinger, the American who died following somatic gene therapy, revealed in his testicular tissue both the presence of the vectors used in the genetic interventions and that of the modified DNA itself (Marshall, 1999).

Ooplasm transplantation

Female infertility can sometimes be due to dysfunctioning ooplasm — the cytoplasm of the egg cells (Cohen et al. 1997). In this case the infertility can be treated in the following way: First, conventional IVF treatment is started. Then the egg cells taken from the infertile woman are injected not only with her partner's sperm, but also with ooplasm from a donor. This means that donor mitochondria can also enter the egg cells. The subsequent procedure is again that of conventional IVF. One advantage of this infertility treatment over other methods is that it does not require the donation of complete egg cells for the fertilization. A woman who is infertile due to defective

---

[8] This risk could be higher in conjunction with so-called *in utero* gene therapy (Anderson, 2000; Frankel & Chapman, 2000).

ooplasm can still have a child from her own egg cells (Cohen et al. 1997; Brenner et al. 2000; Barrit et al. 2001).

In 1996 Jacques Cohen *et al.*, scientists at the *Institute for Reproductive Medicine and Science of Saint Barnabas* in New Jersey, performed such an ooplasm transplantation, resulting in the successful birth of a child (Cohen et al. 1997). Since then, this form of infertility treatment has been successfully implemented another 15 times in New Jersey and approximately 30 times worldwide (Barritt et al. 2001).

Why should these infertility treatments be viewed as a kind of germ line genome modification? After all, the ooplasm transplantation only serves the purpose of successful fertilization and is not directed at any kind of genetic modification to achieve certain characteristics in a future child. Neither does this treatment modify any specific nDNA sequences. The reason is as follows (Bonnicksen, 1998a; Gezondheidsraad, 2001b; Resnik & Langer, 2001). Transplanting ooplasm from the egg cell of a fertile woman to the egg cell of another woman can also lead to mitochondria from the ooplasm donor entering the recipient egg cell. This means that, following successful fertilization, the emerging embryo might have not only mitochondria from its mother, but also mitochondria from the ooplasm donor. Through such treatment the genome of the future child would thus be extended to include — in addition to mtDNA from the mother — foreign mtDNA. This phenomenon is known as 'mitochondrial heteroplasmy' (Barrit et al. 2001).

The results of different genetic tests following ooplasm transplantation aimed at infertility treatment have shown mitochondrial heteroplasmy in the examined cells (Brenner et al. 2000; Barritt et al. 2001). Using appropriate genetic tests, scientists at the *Institute for Reproductive Medicine and Science of Saint Barnabas* registered foreign mtDNA from the ooplasm donors in the blood cells of two one-year old children conceived following ooplasm transplantation (Barritt et al. 2001). The scientists thus felt justified in calling their intervention "the first case of human germ line genetic modification resulting in normal healthy children" (Barritt et al. 2001, 513). Whether it will live up to the optimism behind this title is, however, uncertain. The long-term effects of this infertility treatment on the health of the emerging children are not yet known.

Somatic cell nuclear transplantation

During somatic cell nuclear transplantation the cell nucleus is removed from an egg cell. The nucleus of a somatic cell is then injected in its place. After this, the egg cell is stimulated to start dividing. The chief goal behind current application of this technique in human beings is the harvesting of stem cells, also known as 'therapeutic cloning' (see 5.1.5). However, could also possibly be used in the field of reproduction medicine as an asexual method of reproduction — then termed 'reproductive cloning' — to help absolutely infertile couples have children sharing their own genetic material.

In 2001 scientists from the biotechnological firm *Advanced Cell Technology Inc.* in Massachusetts performed the first published and 'successful' cell nuclear transplantation of this kind. It took place within the framework of experiments to develop stem cell harvesting techniques (Cibelli et al. 2001 & 2002). For these experiments seven young women donated a total of 71 egg cells.[9] In 19 of these egg cells researchers replaced the maternal nuclei with cell nuclei from fibroblasts and cumulus cells from adults.[10] Out of these 19 egg cells just three embryos developed as far as the four or six-cell stage. Since they did not reach the blastocyst stage, they could not be used for the harvesting of ES cells (Cibelli et al. 2001 & 2002).

In the year 2004 Hwang et al., a group of South Korean researchers, were the first to report the derivation of a pluripotent embryonic stem cell line from a cloned human blastocyst. For their experiment 16 volunteers donated 242 oocytes after ovarian stimulation for the express purpose of stem cell derivation after autologous somatic cell nuclear transplantation: the donor's own cumulus cell, isolated from the cumulus-oocyte complex, would be transplanted into the donor's own enucleated oocyte. The protocol Hwang et al. describe produced blastocysts at rates of 19 to 29% (as a percentage of oocytes used). The researchers were only able to derive one embryonic stem cell line from the inner cell mass of 20 cloned embryos. However, they thereby demonstrated the feasibility of generating human ES cells from a somatic cell isolated from a living person (Hwang et al. 2004).

The somatic cell nuclear transplantation technique outlined above can be viewed as a form of germ line genome modification for the following reason: It is true that this technique is not aimed at modifying the genetic material of a future child, and yet the transplantation of genetic material from a somatic cell to an egg cell which has

---

[9] Of these 71 cells, 22 were used for a parthenogenesis experiment: Without being fertilized first, the cells were stimulated with chemicals to start dividing. After 5 days, clearly developing blastoceles could be observed in 6 cell clusters. None of these cell clusters showed a clearly recognizable inner cell mass, however (Cibelli et al. 2001).

[10] The — extremely small — cumulus cells were injected whole into the egg cells.

been stripped of its original nDNA necessarily involves a new nDNA/mtDNA combination. The mtDNA still located in the cytoplasm of the denucleated egg cell is combined with the new genetic material introduced to the egg cell — either new nDNA or, in the case of a whole somatic cell transplantation, additional mtDNA. This means an unequivocal modification of the original genome of the denucleated egg cell (Resnik et al. 2001).

7.1.5 *Potential future germ line genome modifications in human beings*

Future methods of performing germ line genome modifications in human beings cannot be predicted with any certainty. However, various scenarios are already being discussed in the literature. Four example scenarios are outlined below.

Reproductive cloning in human beings

At first sight it would appear logical that a method comparable to reproductive cloning in animals could also — having been modified to agree with human biological insights — be used for the reproductive cloning of human beings (DFG, 2001). And yet various scientific and clinical uncertainties and questions remain as to whether it would really be possible (PHC, 2002). If, for the moment, we assume that it would at least be possible in principle, the actual procedure could be as follows (Fiddler et al. 1999; Hill, 2002; PHC, 2002): Fully differentiated somatic cells from the donor to be cloned would be used as starter cells for the cloning. Their highly-differentiated genetic program could, in the right circumstances, be fully reprogrammed inside the denucleated egg cell (DFG, 2001).

First a cell culture would be prepared from the donated somatic cells. Then they would be starved in order to terminate growth and cell division (Kollek, 1998). It would be vital to ensure that the cell cycles of the cell nucleus being transplanted and of the denucleated egg cell would be synchronized (DFG, 2001; Berardino, 2002; Wolf, 2002). If this were not the case, for example if a cell nucleus taken from a resting cell were to be implanted in a denucleated egg cell which had just begun to prepare its chromosomes for division, then the genetic material of the cell nucleus could be destroyed (DFG, 2001).

The cell nuclear transplantation procedure would commence with the harvesting of a single nucleus from one cell in the culture, using a needle and a micropipette under a microscope. The nucleus of an unfertilized egg cell, which could be either from the same donor or from another donor, would be removed in a similar way. The cell nucleus would then be injected into the denucleated egg cell (DFG, 2001). Instead of injecting the nucleus into the denucleated egg cell, it would also be possible to perform the transplantation by electro-fusion of the complete starter cell with the denucleated egg cell (DFG, 2001). Following successful fusion of the nucleus or whole somatic cell with the denucleated egg cell, an embryo would then begin to develop — in a special culture medium — by way of mitotic cell division.

The nuclear genome of the clone thus emerging would be identical to that of the donor of the starter cells. Regarding the mitochondrial genome, the clone would however differ from the donor, unless the denucleated egg cell was also from the donor of the starter cells and not from a third party (DFG, 2001). Prior to implantation of the clone in the uterus of the future mother, one or more of its cells would be subjected to genetic diagnosis in order to establish the quality and intactness of the cell nuclear genome (PHC, 2002).

It is not yet possible to say whether reproductive cloning in human beings would lead to more, fewer or the same number of anomalies as in animals. It is assumed, however, that the problems arising in connection with the reproductive cloning of other mammals (see 7.1.2) could also occur in conjunction with the reproductive cloning of human beings (Jaenisch & Wilmut, 2001; PHC, 2002). The scientific literature has yet to include any reports describing the successful reproductive cloning of human beings using cell nuclear transplantation. Reports have so far been limited to therapeutic human cloning.

The IVONT protocol

The first scenario involves an intervention which many authors describe as a germ line genome modification (Bonnicksen, 1998a & 1998b; Gezondheidsraad, 2001b; Resnik et al. 2001; Richter et al. 1999; Rubinstein et al. 1995). Its goal is the prevention of a disease caused by a defect in the mtDNA of the mitochondria. The technique used in conjunction with this type of germ line genome modification would principally be as follows: First the cell nucleus would be removed from an egg cell of a woman with a mitochondrial defect. The same would be done with the nucleus of an egg cell from a donor with normally functioning mitochondria. The nucleus from the woman with the mitochondrial defect would then be injected into the denucleated donor egg cell. The resulting egg cell would then be subjected to IVF. The intervention would end with implantation of the fertilized egg cell in the patient's uterus (Rubinstein et al. 1995).

In 1995 Rubenstein *et al.* published a nine-step protocol describing the hypothetical course of such an intervention. Due to the chosen technique outlined above, they called their intervention *in vitro ovum nuclear transplantation* (IVONT). Their IVONT protocol constitutes the first elaborate scenario for a human germ line genome modification ever published.

Rubinstein *et al.* formulated the nine steps as summarized below:

1) The existence of a genetic defect in the patient's mitochondria is diagnosed, for example by examining her family anamnesis, her specific symptoms and by finding an indication of an mtDNA mutation.
2) The patient undergoes genetic counseling.
3) A potential egg cell donor undergoes genetic tests to confirm that her mitochondria are functioning normally.
4) Egg cells are taken from both the patient and the donor — after first synchronizing their menstrual cycles.
5) From the patient's egg cell the cell nucleus is removed and its absolute lack of mitochondria proven. Then the cell nucleus is removed from a donor egg cell.
6) Using IVONT the patient's cell nucleus — free of mitochondria — is injected into the denucleated donor egg cell.
7) The 'IVONT egg cell' undergoes IVF using sperm from the patient's partner, and the resulting 'IVONT zygote' is implanted in the patient's uterus.
8) In order to rule out an mtDNA mutation in the fetus, the pregnant patient undergoes preimplantation diagnosis, chorionic villus sampling or amniocentesis.
9) The newborn child undergoes genetic tests (Rubinstein et al. 1995).

Homologous recombination

The second scenario describes germ line genome modifications using the method of homologous recombination — a process which enables an unwanted genetic sequence to be removed and a new, wanted sequence to take its place in the DNA. Various authors are already speculating about the exact course of such interventions in the future (Capecchi, 2000; Resnik et al. 1999). Present discussion focuses on the two following hypothetical approaches: (1) gene-technological inter- ventions in fertilized egg cells and (2) gene-technological interven- tions in embryonic stem cells (ES cells).

In the first of these approaches, a desired genetic sequence is trans- ferred to a zygote using the mechanism of homologous recombina- tion. Resnik *et al.* (1999) believe the future viability of this approach to hinge on a high success rate and a lack of disturbing side-effects. If the success rate were to be low, a large number of zygotes would be needed for one successful intervention. Many embryos would have to be sorted out and discarded, which would be hard to justify ethically. And in order to exclude undetected defects during the fur- ther development of the embryo, controls would have to be per- formed — such as preimplantation genetic diagnosis (PGD) or amniocentesis. Should a false localization of the new genetic sequence be registered, the embryo would have to be destroyed and the pregnancy terminated (Resnik et al. 1999).

A second theoretical way of manipulating human germ cells using gene technology could, according to Resnik *et al.* (1999), be gene- technological interventions in ES cells (cf. Willgoos, 2001). Here the new, desired genetic sequence would be transferred to the DNA of ES cells — again using the technique of homologous recombination. These pluripotent cells would come from an embryo carrying a genetic defect. The ES cells would first be further cultivated *in vitro* and then genetically manipulated. From the cell culture those cells would then be selected in which the defective genetic sequence has been exactly replaced by the new sequence. Finally, the technique of cell nuclear transplantation would be used to create an embryo from the nucleus of a successfully manipulated ES cell. This embryo would have the same genetic disposition as its donor, with the excep- tion of a new and normally functioning genetic sequence (Resnik et al. 1999; Capecchi, 2000).

Artificial chromosomes

In the last of the three scenarios for potential future germ line genome modifications in human beings, the genome is modified by adding an artificial chromosome — containing a new genetic sequence — to the genome of a fertilized egg cell. This technique could possibly be performed as follows: First, an artificial chromosome would be produced. It would not have its own genes, but instead would be equipped with a series of so-called docking sites, on which — using special enzymes — various desired genetic sequences could be affixed. Once the individual 'cassettes' of the artificial chromosome have been 'filled' in the desired way, the chromosome would then be added to the original genome of a fertilized egg cell. It would thus more or less function as a vehicle for the transferal of various desired genetic sequences to the genome of the egg cell (Campbell & Stock, 2000). Because adding takes place twice — firstly the desired genetic sequences are added to the chromosome, and secondly the chromosome is added to the original set of chromosomes in the egg cell — Campbell & Stock have called this technique "double addition" (Campbell & Stock, 2000, 10).

One advantage of this procedure would be its high level of safety compared with the technique of homologous recombination. With double addition, the original genome would remain untouched. Since this method would also not be particularly invasive, it would probably involve fewer undesirable side-effects. It is conceivable that use of the chromosome vehicle could, in time, lead to not just one genetic sequence but possibly even hundreds being added to the original genome, with all sorts of results. Maybe as the technology is developed further, the individual cassettes filled with new genetic sequences could be activated after a delay. This would open up the possibility of leaving a genetic cassette inactive until the person carrying the artificial chromosome were old enough to decide for him or herself when and if to activate the foreign genetic sequences. Finally, mechanisms could conceivably be developed which would prevent the artificial chromosome from being passed on to any offspring of the carrier. Such mechanisms would be desirable because a set of genetic material implanted in a person as state-of-the-art technology could, one generation later, be outdated and no longer attractive (Campbell & Stock, 2000).

In connection with the generation of transgenic animals, as well as in the context of human somatic gene therapy, research into the development of artificial chromosomes is already underway. If research in this field continues to progress at the current speed, it will not be long before the use of artificial chromosomes for germ line genome modifications in human beings becomes viable.[11] In this context potential realistic future applications are already being discussed. For example, the double addition method could be used in the prevention of AIDS (Campbell & Stock, 2000; cf. Capecchi, 2000; Silver, 1997).

Campbell and Stock explain this possibility as follows: AIDS research to date has shown that the human immune deficiency virus (HIV) causing AIDS is fundamentally geared only towards certain cell types. In particular it infects the T-cells formed by human bone marrow. AIDS researchers are already addressing the development of artificial genes to make T-cells resistant to HIV. If in the future it were possible to implant such genes in the stem cells of a patient's bone marrow, resistant T-cells could form there and prevent the disease from emerging. The double addition method would be interesting here, enabling not only the 'HIV resistance gene' itself to be implanted, but also various regulator sequences. So-called promoters — triggering the transcription of genes — would be a good example. Following further development the HIV resistance gene could then be regulated.[12] Once fully developed, this technique could in principle also be used to prevent other viral diseases — having first been adapted accordingly, of course (Campbell & Stock, 2000).

Campbell and Stock see a further future potential application for germ line genome modifications in the fight against cancer. They have already described in detail a possible use of the double addition method to combat prostate cancer. The approach they have developed would, in their opinion, also be suited to the fight against other types of cancer — again after appropriate adaptation. Finally, they believe artificial chromosomes could be used to prevent neurodegenerative diseases like Alzheimer's, Lou Gehrig's disease or Parkinson's (Campbell & Stock, 2000).

---

[11] The development of cassettes suited to the docking of certain desirable new genetic sequences would so far appear to be more difficult to realize, however (Campbell & Stock, 2000).

[12] It would be desirable if HIV resistance genes were only to be active in cells which can really be affected by HIV — i.e. cells with a CD4 protein on their surface. The following regulation mechanism could be viable: A promotor can only activate a certain gene once a corresponding protein — a so-called transcription factor — has attached itself to it. The idea would be to place the promotor of a CD4 gene before the HIV resistance gene. The promotor of the CD4 gene would only react to the CD4 transcription factor, which in turn is only present in cells which have a CD4 protein on their surface. And so the CD4 promotor would only activate the HIV resistance gene in cells which can actually be affected by HIV (Campbell & Stock, 2000).

7.2 Evaluation of the research field objectives

7.2.1 *Objectives*

Preventing diseases

A major objective behind the research field of germ line genome modification triggering considerable feelings of euphoria is the prevention of various diseases (Campbell & Stock, 2000; Fiddler & Pergament, 1998; Resnik et al. 1999; Resnik & Langer, 2001; Silver, 2000a). Prevention could be conceivable in the form of certain defective genes not being passed on to future generations — meaning they would not contract the otherwise hereditary diseases. In particular, it could be possible to prevent an autosomal recessive genetic defect from being passed on in cases where both parents are homozygous with regard to this defect. Another example would be the possibility of preventing an autosomal dominant genetic defect — e.g. Huntington's disease — from being passed on in cases where one of the parents is homozygous (Capecchi, 2000). In both examples the implementation of germ line genome modifying methods — such as homologous recombination — could possibly prevent a defective gene from being passed on and instead facilitate the implantation of a normally functioning gene in the genome of a future child, and thus prevent the hereditary disease.

Secondly, prevention could occur in the guise of introducing additional genes to the genome of the future child, equipping it to stave off various diseases. This could be the prevention of AIDS, possibly facilitated through appropriate gene technological 'arming' against HIV, or a corresponding 'armor' to fight off cancer (Campbell & Stock, 2000).

Enhancing attributes

The second most important objective behind the research field of germ line genome modification triggering feelings of euphoria is the improvement or enhancement of certain desirable attributes, going beyond the mere prevention of disease (Capecchi, 2000; Engelhardt, 1987; Ennenga, 2000; Hood, 2000; Koshland, 2000; Parens, 2000; Silver, 1997). It is currently impossible to draw an exact line between preventive and enhancing measures. It may be assumed, however, that in the course of ever-advancing germ line genome modification technology interventions will in time become possible which are clearly enhancing.

The geneticist Lee Silver imagined such a development as follows: At first existing technologies would probably be used to modify the germ line genome exclusively in order to prevent diseases which considerably restrict quality of life as early as childhood — e.g. sickle cell anemia or cystic fibrosis. The positive experience gained in this context would quite possibly have a calming effect on any initial public disquiet regarding the new technology. The next step could be an extension of this technology to prevent diseases which do not significantly restrict quality of life until adulthood, for example diabetes, asthma or various kinds of cancer. If this phase were also successful, the next step could be the development of techniques to introduce new genes rendering people immune to severe pathogens like HIV. This stage could also see a first administration of certain new genes — accepted by the public — to improve the health and resilience of children who, without them, would not have had any particular health problems. Many prospective parents would probably be interested in this kind of gene technological intervention, understandably hoping to give their offspring the best genetic material (Silver, 1997; cf. Capecchi, 2000; Koshland, 2000).

In the course of further successful development within this research field, attempts could be made to improve the sensory abilities of a future child. This could be the ability to see infrared light — considerably improving night vision — or the ability to smell as keenly as a dog, for instance. And once the exact influence of genetic material on the cognitive abilities of the human brain were understood, prospective parents could opt to equip their future children with corresponding genes to enhance their intelligence (Silver, 1997). The philosopher Jonathan Glover even believes it possible that human beings could in time use germ line genome modification to overcome emotional failings — like aggression or pugnacity — which in turn could possibly even mean the avoidance of wars (Glover, 1984).

Increasing the reproductive and infertility treatment options available

Further objectives behind the development of methods to modify the genome of the germ line are the extension of both the reproductive methods available and the possible ways of treating infertility. However, these objectives are not considered to be the main causes of utopian euphoria in connection with germ line genome modifications. A detailed ethical analysis of this objective will therefore not be given, instead a few conclusive remarks.

The so-called reproductive cloning method in particular could theoretically constitute a contribution to the first of these objectives (Bouma, 1999; Fiddler et al. 1999; Hershenov, 2000; PHC, 2002; Robertson, 1998; Dooren, 1998; Verzelle, 1998; Willgoos, 2001). The asexual nuclear transplantation method of reproduction would put absolutely infertile heterosexual, as well as homosexual, couples in a position to have children whose genetic material would still be from at least one of the parents (Murphy, 1998; Pence, 1998). It would also enable single males or females to reproduce without needing the genetic material of another person.[13] Reproduction would cease to be the domain of women, with cell nuclear transplantation also enabling men to reproduce.[14] Age would likewise cease to play a crucial role for fertility: reproductive cloning would also enable older women to have children. If we imagine for a moment that the risks associated with reproductive cloning would one day become acceptable, and that its technological application would one day become practicable, then cloning really would contribute to realizing the envisaged objective. However, it is extremely doubtful whether either of these will ever happen.

Assuming that reproductive cloning in humans would unfold similarly to that in other mammals — i.e. that there would be no essential differences — then these doubts can be justified as follows: If reproductive cloning in human beings were to commence now, only a small percentage of the cell nuclear transplantations would actually end in the successful cloning of a human being with normal functions (Berardino, 2002; Jaenisch & Wilmut, 2001; PHC, 2002). A large number of egg cells would be required for just one successful clone. Many women would have to subject themselves to the various risks and unpleasant procedures connected with egg cell donation. Numerous new clones would die whilst still in the uterus. Clones surviving until birth would often display anomalies and/or die soon afterwards. For the mother this would mean repeated and serious risks to her health, as well as all manner of psychological burdens.

---

[13] In the case of a single man this is not strictly true. He would of course still require a donor egg cell and mitochondria.
[14] Here a surrogate mother would be necessary, though.

For reasons of safety and practicability, human reproductive cloning therefore cannot be said to contribute to increasing the reproductive options available at the current time (PHC, 2002).

According to the *Panel on Scientific and Medical Aspects of Human Cloning* (PHC, 2002), in order to facilitate sufficient efficiency and safety in the execution of human reproductive cloning in the long term, at least three conditions must be fulfilled. Firstly, the existing cloning techniques for animals would have to become so advanced that the percentage of anomalies observed in cloned animals — including non-human primates — were at least as low as for other established reproduction techniques. If this could not be achieved, scientists would at least have to prove that human beings are significantly different to animals with regard to their susceptibility to cloning defects. The availability of reproducible data as evidence that successful reprogramming and satisfactory imprinting are possible in animals would be essential. And the mechanisms permitting such success would have to be transparent (PHC, 2002). Secondly, new methods would have to be developed to demonstrate that human preimplantation embryos created with the help of cell nuclear transplantation would function normally with regard to reprogramming and imprinting (PHC, 2002). Thirdly, methods would have to be developed to facilitate effective and comprehensive monitoring of cloned embryos and fetuses in the uterus in order to detect early on any defects connected with the cloning — including alterations in genetic expression or abnormal imprinting (PHC, 2002). At present none of these three conditions can be fulfilled. It is also unsure whether it will ever be possible to fulfill them. As a result, it is currently impossible to say whether, at some time in the future, further development in this research field could contribute to increasing the reproductive options available.

The ooplasm transplantation method could make a contribution to realizing the second objective. After all, it has already been used 'successfully' — in the sense of a successful birth — to treat a certain form of infertility (see 7.1.4). And yet it is too early to say whether this technique will have any unfavorable effects on the health of the children being born. Nothing definitive can yet be said about the long-term medical risks of ooplasm transplantation.

Incidentally, it would have been ethically more cautious to delay ooplasm transplantation experiments on human beings until the procedure had been found — for example following extensive animal research — to be sufficiently safe regarding the long-term risks. The decision to perform ooplasm transplantation as part of infertility treatment was probably influenced by scientific curiosity, however, as well as a desire to fulfill the wishes of prospective parents. These considerations were probably deemed weightier than any desire to protect a future child from potential damage. From an ethical point of view this decision is problematic. The obligation to prevent somebody from coming to harm is greater than the obligation to do good. From an ethical standpoint, the obligation of a physician to protect a future child from harm is greater than his or her obligation to do prospective parents good. Nevertheless, any harm possibly inflicted on the future child was accepted as the price to pay for performing ooplasm transplantation within the framework of infertility treatment. This means that the future child was instrumentalized for the good of its parents and the satisfaction of scientific curiosity, a circumstance which is ethically problematic.

7.2.2 Evaluation

Preventing diseases

In order to achieve a reasonable evaluation of this objective, let us start by assuming that germ line genome modification technology were to be already fully developed. For the sake of argument we shall therefore assume that (1) various germ line genome modification techniques have been proven to prevent diseases, that (2) the risks of implementing these techniques are acceptably low, and that (3) germ line genome modification is sufficiently practicable to render it viable in clinical practice.

Generally speaking, a preventive measure for a particular disease is only desirable if (a) any side-effects associated with the measure are more bearable for the patient than the disease itself, and if (b) the disease cannot be prevented in any other, less complicated way. With regard to germ line genome modification, the first point may be addressed as follows. The diseases which could potentially merit a germ line genome modification involve more or less severe concomitant burdens, depending on the disease in question. They can include chronic pain of varying severity, all manner of dysfunctions, mental retardation and even premature death. One may assume — because the above three conditions are considered to be fulfilled — that a patient's complaints caused by the side-effects associated with the germ line genome modification would be slight. Therefore, various diseases are conceivable which would cause complaints significantly worse than those triggered by the side-effects associated with the preventive measure.

Regarding the second point it may be said that in certain cases there would be no alternative way of preventing the disease and that germ line genome modification would thus represent the only option. This would be the case with an autosomal recessive genetic defect in cases where both parents are homozygous with regard to this defect, or with an autosomal dominant genetic defect — e.g. Huntington's disease — where one of the parents is homozygous (see 7.4.1). Overall, the prevention of diseases does appear to be a desirable objective underlying the research field of germ line genome modification.

Enhancing attributes

As far as an evaluation of the effects to be achieved by enhancing particular attributes is concerned, it should first be established — as touched on above — that there is no clear line marking exactly where interventions preventing disease stop and those enhancing certain attributes begin (Juengst, 1997 & 1998; Parens, 1998). Where the line is drawn depends firstly on one's underlying concept of disease, and secondly on one's view of what constitutes normal (Scully & Rehmann-Sutter, 2001). This ethical analysis does not require a clear demarcation, however. We simply have to remember that there is a grey area between the interventions clearly aimed at preventing disease and those clearly aimed at enhancing attributes. This area would include interventions like the implantation of a new gene to reduce one's cholesterol levels and thus reduce the risk of heart attack.

The possibility of enhancing attributes like intelligence appear at first glance to be desirable. Who would not want to optimize his suboptimal abilities? Is the enhancement of certain attributes really desirable on closer observation, though? A deeper analysis of this question reveals that any enhancement of a particular attribute which appears desirable *prima facie* could have a negative effect on individuals in the longer term (Billings et al. 1999; Peterson, 2001; Roy, 1998). This could be the case if external circumstances should change unfavorably. Strengthening human vision, for example, could cause an extreme and disturbing sensitivity to light if irradiation from the sun were to increase. It is very difficult to estimate whether the attributes given to an individual would make his life easier in the long term. By applying germ line genome modifications aimed at enhancement, one would therefore run the risk of the 'enhanced' individual in time coming to view the effects negatively. It is not as clear as with the prevention of certain diseases that an individual would always experience this kind of germ line genome modification as positive.

It is also difficult to predict how the enhancement of particular, more complex attributes would affect the evolvement of other attributes. How would enhanced intelligence, for example, affect ambition, working ethos, stamina, social skills or self-discipline — all attributes which are equally important for social success (Fukuyama, 2002).[15] If a child's intelligence were to be increased, it could possibly misbehave in school due to boredom at being under-challenged, and then in time turn to criminality.

In the light of these dangers, the use of germ line genome modification to enhance attributes does not appear to be unproblematic. It is important, of course, not to fall into the trap of concentrating exclusively on worst-case scenarios.[16] Every so often a bank is robbed or an estate agent goes bankrupt, and yet that does not lead us to refrain from having money in the bank or buying houses. However, the analysis shows that the question here — of whether the enhancement of attributes using germ line genome modification is fundamentally desirable or not — cannot be answered in a clear affirmative. It is simply not possible to estimate how high the probability would be of external circumstances changing unfavorably, or of negative effects occurring.

7.3 Contribution of the research field to realizing the objectives

7.3.1 *Preventing diseases*

If we assume that germ line genome modification technology were so far advanced that it could be implemented in clinical practice, its application really could mean that the outbreak of certain diseases

---

[15] This is further exacerbated by the problem that it is very difficult to estimate the exact effect of a certain genetic modification within a constellation of genes which, taken together, produces a polygenetic attribute (cf. Hood, 2000).

[16] This sometimes happens in debates about the permissibility of new technologies.

could be avoided. It is not yet certain, however, whether germ line genome modifications will ever be developed to the stage of being successful and practicable methods of preventing diseases. Their development is currently hindered by several key technical obstacles which so far nobody has been able to eliminate, some of which are outlined below.

In connection with the homologous recombination method of modifying the germ line genome — where, ideally, a new gene is introduced to exactly the genetic location previously occupied by a removed defective gene and then firmly integrated within the recipient genome — Resnik et al. (1999) have cited the following four obstacles: Firstly, in order to be able to perform homologous recombination in a zygote, a suitable vector or appropriate method is required to transport the new gene to precisely the genetic location previously occupied by the defective gene. Neither has been developed to date. Practicability would further presuppose a high success rate in order to keep the number of zygotes used as low as possible. For the performance of homologous recombination in embryonic stem cells (ES cells), a method with a high success rate would likewise be required. A high number of starter ES cells would otherwise be required for the successful introduction and integration of just a single new gene in a future child. A method of this efficiency does not exist to date (Resnik et al. 1999).

Secondly, before homologous recombination could successfully be performed in ES cells, various necessary cell manipulation techniques would first have to be improved. They include the routine cultivation and preservation of ES cells, where potential unwanted genetic changes — for example leading to a loss of pluripotency — would also have to be minimized. The technique for removing the cell nucleus from a developing egg cell would also have to be improved. And finally, a sure technique for transplanting genetically manipulated ES cell nuclei would have to be developed, permitting an ES cell nucleus to be physically implanted inside a denucleated egg cell. Such techniques already exist for some animal species, but we cannot simply assume that they would be transferable to human beings (Resnik et al. 1999).

Thirdly, a method would have to be developed to turn back the genetic program of an ES cell nucleus, following its transfer to a denucleated egg cell, to the point of returning the cell nucleus to the developmental stage of a zygote. Only a cell nucleus returned to its totipotent stage could bring about the growth of a complete embryo (Resnik et al. 1999).

And fourthly, genetic tests more precise than any in existence would have to be developed, permitting an exact and reliable analysis of the effect of homologous recombination. The tests currently available to detect genetic defects — e.g. preimplantation diagnostics or prenatal diagnostics, incidentally also involving a certain risk for the embryo — are still not sufficiently error-free. It cannot be guaranteed, for example, that the genotype of the random cell sample taken for biopsy is actually representative of the genotype of the majority of cells in the embryo or fetus. Technical errors cannot be completely ruled out either, meaning that false diagnoses could be made or an existing genetic defect not detected. It therefore seems appropriate to halt the implementation of homologous recombination until there are absolutely precise and reliable ways of diagnosing genetic defects (Resnik et al. 1999).

In connection with the method of modifying the germ line genome presented in the IVONT protocol — where the nucleus of a patient's egg cell is transferred to a denucleated egg cell from a fertile donor — there are still the following issues to be addressed: Firstly there are very few viable animal models to date which could be used as a basis for a risk assessment concerning the application of IVONT to human beings (Gezondheidsraad, 2001b; Richter et al 1999).

Secondly, it is not yet clear how the patient nucleus and the denucleated donor egg cell would react to the transplantation. It is unclear, for example, whether the removal of an endogenous nucleus and the subsequent implantation of an exogenous nucleus would have a negative influence on the further development of the egg cell (Gezondheidsraad, 2001b).

Thirdly, the absolutely mitochondria-free extraction of a nucleus from an egg cell of the patient — which is necessary if IVONT treatment is to be successful — cannot yet be guaranteed. The technology for this does not exist yet. It is also unclear how the egg cell nucleus would react to the rinsing procedure required to ensure its complete freedom from mitochondria (Gezondheidsraad, 2001b; Richter, 1999).

Fourthly, it is conceivable that there could be compatibility problems between the nDNA and mtDNA (Gezondheidsraad, 2001b; Richter, 1999). If the chromosomal and mitochondrial genes were somehow to be incompatible, the possibility of auto-antibodies developing as a reaction to the complete cytoplasm exchange could not be ruled out (Richter, 1999). Natural fertilization also involves a high number of mtDNA and nDNA combinations, but we do not yet know how often compatibility problems occur. However, it is probable that compatibility problems would not occur any more frequently using the IVONT technique than as a result of natural fertilization (Gezondheidsraad, 2001b).

Finally, we have no way of yet knowing how the method described in the IVONT protocol would affect the development of the emerging embryo. Since the first steps of the fertilization process are particularly crucial for further embryonic development, a close observation of the effects of IVONT on the young embryo or fetus, as well as the newborn child, would be indicated in this context (Richter, 1999).

Regarding germ line genome modifications using artificial chromosomes, there are also various technical obstacles to be overcome. Research into the development of artificial chromosomes is already underway, but the development of suitable 'docking stations' which could be filled with various genes and corresponding regulators seems to be technically quite complicated (Campbell & Stock, 2000). Moreover, the knowledge required to construct a defect-free and safely functioning artificial chromosome within the genome of a future child is far from complete (Campbell & Stock, 2000). Neither is there a mechanism yet available to prevent the artificial chromosome from being inherited by the next generation (Campbell & Stock, 2000).

At the current time we can only speculate as to whether the cited obstacles will ever be overcome in the future. Consequently, we cannot yet know whether in the long term germ line genome modifications would contribute to realizing the abovementioned objective — i.e. whether they will ever be developed to the point of preventing diseases in clinical practice. Many authors are already convinced, however, that in the future we will have suitable technologies enabling germ line genome modifications to be implemented (Billings, 1999; Capecchi, 2000; Campbell & Stock, 2000; Fiddler & Pergament, 1998; Silver, 1997; Wadman, 1998; Zimmerman, 2000).

7.3.2 Enhancing attributes

If we assume for a moment that the abovementioned technical problems surrounding the development of techniques enabling germ line genome modifications to be implemented sufficiently safely were all solved, and that germ line genome modifications aimed at preventing diseases could begin, the possibility of the same techniques being used to enhance certain human attributes cannot then be excluded. The enhancement of simple, monogenetically regulated attributes does appear to be more easily realizable than enhancement which is aimed specifically at polygenetic attributes (Willgoos, 2001). And yet, since we do not know how likely it is that the technical requirements will all be met in the future, the contribution of germ line genome modifications to enhancing certain attributes will have to be left open for now.

7.4 Ethical problems

7.4.1 *Problems of responsible development and appropriate use*

Risks

In the ethical debate about germ line genome modifications, the risks involved are an important — for some authors the most important — discussion point (Pence, 2000). There are different risks conceivable in connection with the various potential ways of modifying the germ line genome, primarily depending on the course of the genetic inter-vention performed. The risks involved in an endeavor to use the homologous recombination technique to replace a defective gene with a new one, for example, would depend on whether the replace-ment went smoothly or not. If the new gene replacing the defective one were to function as envisaged, and were it not to hinder the func-tions of any other genes, then the potential risks would essentially be limited to the occurrence of side-effects. And these could even be negligible. By contrast, were the homologous recombination to fail, much greater risks would be involved. The new gene could nega-tively influence other genes within the recipient genome and damage cell function. This could in turn lead to not only the genetically manipulated embryo itself, but also the generations to follow devel-oping severe deformities or even new, unknown genetic diseases. In addition, the effects of germ line genome modifications, unlike most medical interventions currently practiced, would be extensive, per-manent and systemic. The manipulated genome would influence the entire development of a human being, his growth, regulation of his various cells, etc. (Resnik et al. 1999).

Besides the course of the germ line genome modification interven-tion, the extent of the intervention could also influence the degree of risk involved. The manipulation of several genes would appear to involve a higher risk than that of a single gene, for example. The timing of the genetic expression or the degree of interaction between the molecules produced by the new gene and other molecules could also influence the level of risk involved in a particular intervention (Resnik et al. 1999).

A completely different kind of risk would be involved in the use of manipulated viruses or bacteria to transfer a new gene to the recipient genome. It would be conceivable, for instance, that during their preparation new, unknown pathogens could unintentionally develop. These new pathogens could be in danger of causing huge devastation to the human species or of destroying entire ecosystems (Resnik et al. 1999).

In order to facilitate a solid estimate of the risks involved in germ line genome modification, the conduction of various animal experiments is indicated (Wert, 1999; Koshland, 2000) Extensive clinical trials would then be necessary for the collection of sufficient data permitting conclusions to be drawn about those potential risks. Such extensive data material could be a long time in coming, however. A well-founded assessment of the concomitant risks of germ line genome modification is therefore impossible at the present time (Resnik et al. 1999).

It is already clear, however, that the risks involved in any method of modifying the germ line genome would partly depend on the following factors: Firstly, it would matter whether the intervention would modify just the mtDNA, just the nDNA or the original combination of the two. Secondly, it would be significant whether the introduction of transgenes to germ line cells occurred *ex vivo* or *in vivo*. Thirdly, it should be established whether the protocol of a chosen intervention included a special selective measure to increase the probability of actually achieving the envisaged modification in the germ line genome. This measure could be a mechanism which only selected those genetically modified cells for survival which actually contained the desired modification in their genome, causing all deviating cells to die. Fourthly, it would be important to establish the extent of the probability that the selected method could bring about an unintended genetic modification in the germ line genome instead of the desired one, or in addition to it. Finally, it should be ascertained whether the method contained a kind of safety mechanism to reverse the triggered modification in the genome, should it go wrong (Resnik et al. 2001).

Informed consent

Changes in the germ line genome could have potentially severe consequences for the offspring of the genome carrier (Fowler et al. 1989; Lappé, 1991). Because of this, the ethical debate is addressing the extent to which it should be deemed problematic that the offspring would necessarily be unable to consent to the intervention (Billings, 1999; Lappé, 1991; Moseley, 1991; Munson & Davis, 1992). Some authors view this lack of consent as an argument against the implementation of germ line genome modifications (Poliwoda, 1992).

However, the principle of informed consent — that these authors refer to — only applies to people who are in a position to give their consent. In case of germ line genome modifications the prerequisites for the ability to give consent are not fulfilled, neither for the emerging embryo, nor for the future generations. At the moment of intervention in the genetic material, no individuals exist whose consent could possibly be obtained (Birnbacher, 1994; Munson & Davis, 1992). This means that a physician performing a germ line genome modification would be released from the medical obligation to obtain informed consent beforehand.[17] The problem of future generations not giving their informed consent to germ line genome modifications is therefore literally a pseudo-problem. The fundamentally impossible — obtaining consent from future generations regarding decisions which will affect them — cannot be an ethical prerequisite.

If we take the issue as being a problem of responsibility towards future generations, however, then it begins to make more sense. The fundamental impossibility of obtaining consent from future generations does not mean that we do not have to account to them for our actions at all (cf. Agius & Busuttil, 1998a & 1998b; Frankel & Chapman, 2000; McGee, 2000; Salvi, 2001).

An approach to incorporating responsibility for future generations into actual decision-making processes was put forward by Agius (1998a & 1998b). His idea was as follows: The interests of future generations could be represented by so-called guardians. In various debates about decisions affecting the future, these guardians would

---

[17] With regard to the embryo, an ethical prerequisite for treatment could be *proxy consent*. A rule could be established whereby no medical interventions may be performed without the direct next-of-kin (in the case of an embryo its parents) being comprehensively informed and then giving their free consent by proxy (cf. Moseley, 1991).

assume the function of advocates for the generations to come (Agius, 1998a & 1998b). This idea of having advocates to speak for future generations does still have some intransparencies, however. Should these guardians belong to governmental organizations, non-governmental organizations or maybe the United Nations? Ideally, should they come professionally from a scientific, legal or political background (Agius & Busuttil, 1998a & 1998b)? The idea of setting up guardians does seem to merit further debate and clarification, however (cf. Mallia & Have, 2003).

Germ line genome modifications as superfluous

A further problem discussed in the ethical literature regarding germ line genome modifications is that of whether or not these interventions amount to superfluous treatment (cf. Billings, 1999; Fowler et al. 1989; Hubbard, 2000; Zimmerman, 1991). We cannot analyze this problem without first asking ourselves when a new method of treatment can be regarded as superfluous. It is superfluous if, firstly, an existing method of treatment can achieve the same result and, secondly, this existing method is equally or even less complex than the new method.

Regarding these two 'superfluousness criteria', in various cases more simple measures for the prevention of a disease other than germ line genome modification do come to mind. If, for example, both parents are heterozygous carriers of a recessive defective gene, then IVF could be performed, followed by a preimplantation genetic diagnosis. Only those embryos not displaying the genetic defect would then be implanted in the uterus (Fowler et al. 1989; Berger & Gert, 1991; Resnik & Langer, 2001). This method would not only successfully prevent such diseases; it would also be quite easy to perform. In contrast, germ line genome modification is in itself very complicated. Moreover, it would also have to be followed by a preimplantation genetic diagnosis in order to test whether the genetic defect has really been eliminated. Other more successful and simultaneously simpler alternatives to germ line genome modification would in many cases be the adoption of a child, the use of donor gametes or various postnatal treatments (Hubbard, 2000; Resnik et al. 1999; Resnik & Langer, 2000; Schroeder-Kurth, 2000).

There are cases, however, in which germ line genome modification would be the only option, or the least complex option of those available, in order to achieve a particular goal. Resnik et al. (1999) have cited four such cases: Firstly, germ line genome modifications could help in cases where both parents are homozygous for a certain genetic defect. Using germ line genome modification, a normally functioning gene could be introduced to the genome of the future child via the mechanism of homologous recombination. Here, a preimplantation genetic diagnosis followed by embryo selection would not be a suitable alternative way of preventing the disease from emerging (Resnik et al. 1999).

Secondly, germ line genome modifications would be indicated in cases where a couple would like to change various non-linked, monogenetic attributes in the genome of their future child. Here too, a preimplantation genetic diagnosis followed by embryo selection would not usually be a suitable alternative: A large number of embryos would have to be screened in order to find the desired combination of genes (Resnik et al. 1999).

Thirdly, germ line genome modifications could be helpful in cases where a polygenetic attribute is to be modified. The corresponding techniques — e.g. homologous recombination — would permit several different genes to be introduced to the DNA. For the same reasons as with the second case above, a preimplantation genetic diagnosis followed by embryo selection would not be a suitable alternative (Resnik et al. 1999).

Fourthly, germ line genome modification would enable completely new genes to be introduced to the germ line. If parents wished their future child to have one or more genes not in their own genomes, or certain genes from an organism of another species, for example, this wish could only be fulfilled using germ line genome modification. Examples of such desirable new genes could be one reducing the probability of developing cancer or one — possibly stemming from another species — immunizing the future child against certain pathogens (Resnik et al. 1999).[18]

In a more detailed list, full of subtle nuances, Resnik and Langer (2001) go so far as to name eleven different areas in which germ line

---

[18] When a completely new gene is introduced to the genome of a human being, homologous recombination cannot really take place since a gene is not being swapped for a replacement gene. In order to be able to perform homologous recombination anyway (this mechanism enables the new gene to become firmly integrated in the recipient chromosome, as desired), Resnik et al. suggest equipping the new gene with base sequences which are homologous to DNA sequences in a particular part of the recipient genome. Resnik et al. call this part of the DNA the 'transgene acceptor site' (Resnik et al. 1999).

genome modifications represent either the only option or a comparably less complicated option in the quest to realize a particular goal. The list includes the treatment of a woman with dysfunctioning ooplasm desiring a child with her own genetic material. This wish could only be fulfilled with the help of an ooplasm transplantation — which in turn would most likely entail a germ line genome modification. It also includes the use of germ line genome modification to prevent a disease stemming from a genetic defect in the maternal mitochondria from being passed on to offspring. And a third inclusion is somatic cell nuclear transplantation used as a method of reproduction in cases where a couple are absolutely infertile but still wish to have a child bearing the genetic material of at least one of its parents (Resnik & Langer, 2001).

It is very difficult to say whether germ line genome modification really will represent the simplest — or only — method of achieving the medical goals envisaged in the cited cases in the future. In time a simpler, alternative method could emerge. It will, after all, probably be some time before it is clear whether certain techniques used to modify the germ line genome really would be effective with regard to the medical goals listed. The same is true for the concomitant risks of a clinical application, which would have to be ethically acceptable first, as well as the practicability of the method, which would also have to be viable. It is quite possible that by the time all this has come to be realized, simpler and more efficient methods will be available which are not presently conceivable.

It is also doubtful whether the cost/benefit ratio of germ line genome modifications could ever become attractive enough to secure these treatments a sufficiently high ranking above other alternative methods in the light of steady cuts to healthcare budgets (cf. Juengst, 1991). It should be noted at this point, however, that germ line genome modifications would not necessarily be more expensive than alternative methods in the long term. Some of these alternative methods — e.g. somatic gene therapy — would have to be performed anew for each coming generation. To date, the alternatives do appear to be cheaper than germ line genome modifications as stand-alone solutions. But if we take into account that they would have to be repeated for each new generation, the alternative methods could even turn out *summa summarum* to be more expensive (Walters, 1986; Zimmerman, 1991).

In summary, there appear at present to be some situations in which germ line genome modification would represent either the only or the least complex way of achieving a particular goal (Resnik et al. 1999; Resnik & Langer, 2001; Zimmerman, 1991). Consequently, germ line genome modifications cannot be viewed as superfluous. The actual implementation of such technologies in clinical practice does, however, still seem very hypothetical. And it remains unclear for now whether the prerequisites for their implementation will ever be fulfilled.

7.4.2 *Problems intrinsically linked with the technology*

The destruction of embryos

The ethical problem of embryo destruction would accompany any further development of germ line genome modification technology. It would already arise in conjunction with the numerous embryo experiments required just for the development of sufficiently safe germ line genome modification techniques (Billings, 1999; Enquetekommission, 1988; Poliwoda, 1992; Schroeder-Kurth, 2000; Sorg, 1992).

Germ line genome modifications in clinical practice would also entail the destruction of embryos. An intervention would be followed by a preimplantation genetic diagnosis to test the success of the treatment. The cells taken for this diagnosis (blastomeres) would probably still be totipotent, however.[19] Under the right circumstances, they could therefore develop into a complete organism. This means that such cells can be viewed as embryos. The diagnostic method performed following a germ line genome modification would necessarily involve the destruction of a blastomere, and therefore of an embryo.

Elsewhere the author has already justified why an embryo should be attributed full protection from the start of its existence (cf. 5.4.2). This would mean, however, that the destruction of embryos necessarily involved in germ line genome modifications would be reason enough to prohibit such interventions (Poliwoda, 1992).

The following comment should be made at this point. In this analysis it is assumed that in order to detect a potential genetic defect, a totipotent cell would have to be removed and in the course of the ensuing examination destroyed, even in the future. This is not

---

[19] We do not yet know for certain whether cells at the 6-10 cells stage — the developmental stage at which blastomere biopsy is performed — are actually still totipotent (Wert, 1999).

absolutely certain, however. It is — at least theoretically — conceivable that in time a new form of embryonic genetic diagnosis will be developed, which would not necessarily involve the destruction of a totipotent cell. Two possible ways of performing genetic diagnostics on embryos without destroying totipotent cells are already being looked into. The first involves using the polar body from within an egg cell for the genetic tests. This method would have the disadvantage that only the maternal genome of the future embryo can be examined. The second possibility uses cells at a later stage of development for the genetic tests. They are no longer totipotent and can thus not develop into a complete embryo. This second method has the disadvantage that the implantation of incubated blastocysts in the uterus is not nearly as successful (Richter & Schmidt, 1999).

To date there are no adequate ways of performing preimplantation genetic diagnostics on an embryo without destroying a totipotent cell. And since, as has already been said, it is not clear whether this will ever become possible in the future, the ethical problem of embryo destruction remains for now a problem intrinsically linked with the technology of germ line genome modification.

A right to non-modified genetic material

A problem often debated in conjunction with germ line genome modification is the existence of a moral right to a non-modified genome (cf. Wachter, 1993; Mauron & Trevoz; 1991; Mundson & Davis, 1992; Nolan, 1991 Daele, 1985). Accordingly, everybody would have this moral right. Modifications to the germ line genome would violate this right (Enquetekommission, 1988; Lunshof, 1994; Poliwoda, 1992).

In order to assess whether human beings really do have a moral right to non-modified genes, we first have to interpret the term 'moral right'. Our answer will depend on that interpretation. According to Feinberg (1994), a moral right is neither the result of certain legislation, nor the product of social convention; its foundations are independent of both. This means that a moral right can still exist when refuted by legislation or social convention. Based on the correlation of rights and obligations, each moral right for one person corresponds to a moral obligation for another person, and *vice versa* (Feinberg, 1994). Thus, if there really were a moral right to a non-modified genetic inheritance, this would automatically imply a moral obligation not to carry out germ line genome modifications in human beings.

Looked at more closely, however, this moral right, as well as its corresponding moral obligation, appear questionable. The possession of a genome 'as nature intended' no longer seems automatically desirable. We only need to think of cases where the genome contains defects which can lead to severe hereditary diseases, like Huntington's disease or cystic fibrosis. In such cases it would appear to be less in the interests of the carrier of the genome to insist on his right to it and to leave it untouched, than to make the effort to eliminate the genetic defect contained therein.

Likewise, the moral obligation not to carry out any germ line genome modifications in human beings would lead to doubtful consequences. Let us assume for a moment that a particular germ line genome modification technique could in the future really help to prevent certain diseases. And let us also assume that the risks associated with the clinical application of this technique were acceptable, and that its clinical application were practicable. Then we can think of several cases where a modification of the genome would even be ethically indicated. If, for example, both parents were to be homozygous with regard to a particular defect, then the possibility of this defect being passed on to a future child could only be prevented by modifying the genome of that child. The same goes for the passing on of an autosomal recessive genetic defect or an autosomal dominant genetic defect, where one of the parents were homozygous. Only a germ line genome modification could help. A moral obligation not to carry out any germ line genome modifications in human beings would prohibit all these interventions which — under the aforementioned circumstances — would even be ethically desirable.

The moral right to non-modified genes, plus the corresponding moral obligation not to perform any germ line genome modifications in human beings, thus seem to lead to the bizarre consequence of one being morally obliged to refrain from an action which is simultaneously ethically desirable. This is thus a *reductio ad absurdum*. For this reason, a moral right to non-manipulated genetic material as defined above cannot exist (cf. Tännsjö, 1993).

The alteration of personal identity

A further argument against germ line genome modification concerns personal identity. It is seen as problematic that, following a germ line genome modification, a person would no longer be identical to the person before the modification (Enquetekommission, 1988). For an assessment of this argument we need to take a closer look at what exactly is meant by personal identity. Personal identity is given when a person (P_1) at a certain moment in time (T_1) is identical to another person (P_2) at another moment in time (T_2). Put more precisely, this is so-called diachronous personal identity, to be distinguished from so-called synchronous personal identity (Gordijn, 1996). In the ethical argument addressed here, diachronous personal identity is presumed to be morally worthy of respect and protection. A gene technological intervention in the germ line would represent an alteration of this identity and thus an immoral action.

This raises the following difficulty: In principle, a person can only be subjected to an alteration destroying his or her identity if, at the time of that altering intervention, a person can already be said to exist. At what point in human development can we begin to speak of a person? In the argument addressed it is assumed that a person exists at the time of the germ line genome modification, i.e. that a gamete, a zygote or an embryo at the two to eight-cell stage constitutes a person. The precise point in ontogenetic development from which a human being can be viewed as a person has been extensively debated in bioethics. The standpoints involved in this debate range from the moment of conception to selected moments after the birth. Consensus does exist, however, about gametes, which cannot be viewed as persons. The above problem can therefore be said to be non-existent for interventions involving gametes.

For our further analysis we shall therefore concentrate on genetechnological interventions involving zygotes or embryos at the two to eight-cell stage. Taking the view — for the sake of argument — that an embryo is a person from the moment of its conception (Eijk, 1997; Jochemsen, 1989; Kreeft, 1990; Pellegrino, 2000), is the identity of an embryo at the two to eight-cell stage — viewed here as a person — altered by intervening in its germ line genome? This can only be answered by first gaining more information about what exactly constitutes diachronous personal identity, i.e. the circumstances under which a person P_1 existing at a moment in time T_1 can be considered identical to a person P_2 existing at a moment in time T_2. Only then can we analyze whether interventions which modify the germ line genome really would also modify personal identity.

Various criteria for diachronous personal identity have been developed over the past few decades, especially by Anglo-Saxon philosophers. Some of these criteria refer to physical characteristics, and others to mental attributes (Gordijn, 1996). Since, at least according to scientific findings to date, an embryo at the two to eight-cell stage does not possess any mental attributes — not even a nervous system, which would permit mental attributes, has begun to develop yet — not one of the criteria for diachronous personal identity based on mental attributes is applicable here. Of the criteria based on physical characteristics, all those which presuppose the existence of a brain can be discounted. The remaining physical criteria view the identity — or continuity of the functional organization — of the body belonging to a person P_1 with the body of a person P_2 as a criterion for whether these two persons are identical. The strict criterion of diachronous physical identity to determine personal identity is problematic, however. It would mean that no adult were personally identical to the child he or she once was, as the adult body is no longer identical to the body of childhood. With this in mind, nearly all authors participating in the debate about criteria for diachronous personal identity reject the strict physical criterion.

In order to circumnavigate this problem, the strict physical criterion has been modified to render as a prerequisite for diachronous personal identity no longer the diachronous identity of the body, but merely the continuity of its functional organization. This 'revised physical criterion' now reads: "A person P_2 at a moment in time T_2 is the same person as a person P_1 at a moment in time T_1 if the body of P_2 at T_2 is the result of a series of gradual exchanges of material (retaining the continuity of the functional organization of the body) within the body of P_1 at T_1" (Gordijn, 1996). Since the continuity of the functional organization of the embryo in question would definitely be retained in connection with the application of germ line genome modifications, its diachronous personal identity would not — following the revised physical criterion — be changed by such interventions.

In summary, the problem of altering diachronous personal identity turns out to be non-existent. It is not applicable to gene-technological interventions in human gametes, as gametes cannot be regarded as persons. Regarding gene-technological interventions in zygotes or embryos at the two to eight-cell stage, the problem only exists if the zygote or early embryo — following the conceptionalistic view — is already viewed as a person. In this case an intervention altering the germ line genome would not alter diachronous personal identity — following the revised physical criterion. Following the strict physical criterion, a germ line genome modification could be viewed as altering the diachronous personal identity of a zygote or embryo at the two to eight-cell stage. Following this strict criterion, however, diachronous personal identity would change with every cell division of the organism anyway. Consequently, a further alteration to diachronous personal identity, bearing in mind these continual changes happening anyway, would no longer be of particular ethical significance. Moreover, the strict criterion is rejected by most current authors. Overall, the problem of altering diachronous personal identity is revealed to be a pseudo-problem (cf. Holtug & Sandøe, 1996).

Human dignity

An argument frequently discussed in the literature is the violation of human dignity which could potentially accompany germ line genome modifications (cf. Birnbacher, 1994; Council of Europe, 1982; Enquetekommission, 1988; Munson & Davis, 1992; Sutton 1995; Daele, 1985).

The question of whether germ line genome modifications really would constitute a violation of human dignity — as some authors maintain (Convention on Human Rights, 1988; Enquetekommission, 1988; Poliwoda, 1992; Sutton 1995; Daele, 1985) — depends on the interpretation of human dignity. When the human dignity argument is raised, however, there is rarely an explanation of how it is to be comprehended (see e.g. Convention on Human Rights, 1988). And yet some clarity would appear necessary as a whole range of different views exists as to what this term signifies (cf. Hailer & Ritschl, 1996).

The term human dignity, or *dignitas humana*, has only been in existence *expressis verbis* since the Enlightenment, but the concept behind it has been around for much longer (cf. Spiegelberg, 1970). The origins of the term dignity are to be found in the Latin term *dignitas*, which was only used in connection with selected lofty social functions. The idea of a human dignity fundamentally inherent to every human being — independently of social status — primarily stems from early Christian theology, but was already anticipated in Stoic philosophy (Bayertz, 1996; Hailer & Ritschl, 1996). This Christian thought was founded on the idea of man being created in God's image. The influential notion that every human being possesses a certain dignity represents an important contribution to Western ethics by Christianity. Over the course of time the original Christian view of human dignity has developed in various directions, however.

As an illustration of the range covered by these views, two important traditional lines of thought regarding human dignity are worth mentioning: the humanistic tradition and that of the Enlightenment. The former may be represented by Giovanni Pico della Mirandola (1463-1494), the latter by Immanuel Kant (1724-1804).

Pico believed that mankind is the only species on Earth upon whom God did not bestow an unchangeable nature from the outset. Man's dignity lies in the possibility granted to him of shaping himself into what he would like to be (Mirandola, 1486). On the basis of this concept of human dignity there is no need to examine whether germ line genome modifications would violate human dignity. According to Pico, human dignity is something human beings are fundamentally equipped with during God's creation. As such it is principally non-violable.

Kant's view of human dignity is very different. He distinguishes between man as a being of reason on the one hand, and beings without reason on the other. For Kant, the latter are things, and as such only have a value to the extent that they can serve as instruments to attain certain ends. In contrast, man is an end in his own right. As a being equipped with reason, his nature possesses an absolute inner value. In Kant's view, human dignity is embodied by precisely this circumstance. Since every human being is bestowed by nature with an absolute inner value and thus dignity, man should therefore regard not only himself but also all his fellow human beings as ends in themselves, and act accordingly. According to Kant, no human being may use another exclusively as a means to achieve certain ends. Any such instrumentalization of a human being would violate his inherent dignity (Kant, 1785 & 1788).

Following on from this, not every application of techniques to modify the germ line genome would directly signify a violation of human dignity. It is at least conceivable that a modest intervention in the germ line genome would not signify any instrumentalization, merely preventing a particular disease (see 7.2.1). Taking Kant's concept of human dignity, not all germ line genome modifications would infringe upon human dignity. This would mean that all categorically negative evaluations of germ line genome modification which refer to a violation of human dignity in Kant's interpretation — as developed by e.g. Sutton (1995) — would have to be disqualified.

Poliwoda (1992), who also argues on the basis of Kant's conception of dignity, particularly views the instrumentalization of embryos accompanying germ line genome modifications as a violation of human dignity. And yet Kant's concept of human dignity is only applicable to man as a reasonable being. It is thus questionable whether Kant's concept of human dignity can really be applied to embryos. Adhering strictly to Kant, it would maybe be more correct to agree with Heller (2000), who argues that germ line genome modifications cannot infringe upon human dignity. At the moment when the germ line genome modification would take place, a bearer of such dignity would not yet exist.

These deliberations do not imply, however, that it would be fundamentally impossible to violate human dignity in Kant's sense of the phrase by modifying the germ line genome. It would certainly be violated if serious attempts were made to alter the genome of a future individual so comprehensively as to 'program' it for the assumption of certain functions in society, for example. This kind of germ line genome modification would definitely constitute an instrumentalization of human life and thus a violation of human dignity (cf. Birnbacher, 1994).

Playing God

Authors who bring up the 'playing God' argument believe that man has no right to alter the human genetic material created by divine power in a way that the changes could be inherited by children. In their opinion, germ line genome modifications — especially enhancing interventions — constitute a wanton hubris towards God and thus an immoral alteration of the rational and divine order of things (Kass, 1985; Lunshof, 1994; Messer, 1999; Poliwoda, 1992; Ramsey, 1970).

The 'playing God' argument has already been analyzed as an objection to bioelectronic interventions in human beings (see 6.4.2). As with this other field, the use of this argument in connection with germ line genome modification is not without its problems. The very foundations of this argument are problematic. They presuppose the existence of a Creator God, for which there is no generally acknowledged, rational justification. The assumption that a Creator God exists depends far more on one's beliefs than on the results of intellectual debate.

Assuming for a moment, however, that a Creator God does exist, further development of this argument still remains problematic. A reference to God could be the basis for all kinds of argument. Freundel (2000), for example, formulates the following version: Because God created man with a free will, He would be committing an error if He were to forbid him to carry out germ line genome modifications — assuming they could be performed safely. After all, God would then be robbing prospective parents of their free will to decide about germ line genome modifications (Freundel, 2000).

Of course this argument is fundamentally flawed, but the circumstance that authors are able to develop all manner of arguments, on the basis that God is assumed to exist, both for and against germ line genome modifications raises the question of whether any clear indications in a particular direction exist at all, for example that alterations to the human germ line genome really would constitute an overstepping of the boundaries established by God for human action, and thus an infringement of the 'divine order'. In summary, the 'playing God' argument in its theological version seems difficult to uphold. Firstly, the search for rational justification of the existence of a Creator God remains an unsolved intellectual problem. Secondly, even if the existence of a Creator God is assumed, it is still unclear just why germ line genome modifications should in particular not be permissible.

There is another, non-theological version of the 'playing God' argument, which stresses that we simply have too little knowledge and discretion at present to contemplate implementing germ line genome modifications responsibly (Billings, 2000). This is why germ line genome modifications would constitute hubris. For now this version of the argument can be underlined insofar as it can be seen as a warning not to underestimate the complexity of the problems surrounding germ line genome modifications. It can make us aware that we should not overestimate our own wisdom regarding responsible application of what is still pretty basic knowledge.

The human genotype 'as nature intended'

In the opinion of some authors, germ line genome modifications would infringe upon the natural order of things and are therefore to be viewed as ethically problematic (Jonas, 1985; Lunshof, 1994; Poliwoda, 1992; Sorg, 1992). They believe that no human being has the right to intervene in the natural evolutionary order of things if this would permanently change the human genetic material accomplished by evolution thus far. Such interventions in the human germ line would violate the holiness of nature and its intrinsic value. As a result, the freedom of action of one human being must not be allowed to extend to manipulating the genotype of another human being using germ line gene technology.

The problem described above is based on the assumption that the genotype of each human individual possesses an intrinsic value. This is, however, debatable. Does every human genome brought forth by nature — as opposed to 'culture' or 'technology' — really possess a value *per se*?

To answer this, we first need to distinguish between the ontogenetic level of the human individual and the phylogenetic origins of mankind. In the light of the severe hereditary diseases that can befall a human being — such as cystic fibrosis, Huntington's disease or muscular dystrophy — it is doubtful whether, regarding an *individual* human life, every human genome brought forth by nature can be said to possess a value *per se*.

The *phylogenetic* development of mankind has been driven on by the circumstance that, as a result of natural selection, only those organisms have survived whose genetic constellations have by chance, at any one time, proved suitable for successful reproduction in the everchanging circumstances. Organisms not having at their disposal the corresponding favorable attributes at a time of environmental change have slowly but surely been sifted out. The human genome, comprehended as being the genome of the species 'mankind', is in the opinion of modern biologists purely the result of the effects of natural selection and, as such, the product of a contingent process.

With this in mind, it is true to say that the human genome has definitely proved itself to be of instrumental worth. After all, it has enabled the species 'mankind' to survive in contingent circumstances. These deliberations do not rule out the possibility, however, that man could create genomes which would be even more valuable than those brought forth by nature. Examples of such potentially more valuable 'artificial' genomes would be ones which no longer contain defects causing certain hereditary diseases. If, in conjunction with germ line genome modifications, the values of altered human genomes, created by man, and unaltered human genomes, brought forth by nature, were to be assessed, it would not be a foregone conclusion that the natural genomes would achieve the better result (cf. Engelhardt, 1987).

As a result of the above, arguing that gene-technological interventions in the human germ line would sacrifice the intrinsic value of natural genomes and thus be morally reprehensible would not appear to be particularly sound. At least in some cases — for example where a genome is revealed to contain severe genetic defects — it should therefore be deliberated whether, in a direct comparison of their values, the modified germ line genome would not be worth more than the genome 'as nature intended'.

7.4.3 Undesirable effects in the longer term

Geneticization

A process can currently be observed within our society whereby human beings and human behavior are increasingly being presented and explained from a genetic vantage point. This growing influence of genetics has been the basis of several studies. Nelkin und Lindee (1995), for example, examined the effects of modern genetics on the mass culture of Western society. The results of their study show that diverse references to DNA, genes and genetics appear in the various media — be it films, television, the press, comics or advertisements. More and more frequently, the everyday media touch on the idea that the essence of man, his true self, is somehow or other to be found in his genes. According to Nelkin und Lindee, it is almost as though genes have taken the place of the seemingly now old-fashioned soul, have now become the core of human identity. It is as if the self were gradually being reduced to a molecular entity, with man in all his complexity being treated as equivalent to his genes. Lippman (1991) also maintains that the differences between individuals are steadily being reduced to their different genotypes, a process she refers to as 'geneticization'. In more general terms, geneticization can be defined as a process whereby an increasing number of phenomena pertaining to human existence are being drawn into the realm of genetics (Have, 2001; Zwieten & Have, 1998).

The further development and potential application of germ line genome modifications could spur on this process (cf. Hubbard, 2000). If germ line genome modification technology really were to be developed successfully, in the eyes of many this would be a great victory for genetics. The success of germ line genome modifications could then be viewed as confirmation of a kind of genetic reductionism. In such a scenario it is not inconceivable that genetic approaches to explaining phenomena and solving problems would dominate even more than they already do at present. This one-sided orientation could lead to health policy becoming increasingly directed towards genetic detection and intervention, whilst neglecting other potential — such as psychological, social, cultural or physical — causative factors. In addition, there would be the danger of certain social problems, like criminality, being increasingly attributed to measurable biological dimensions — such as genetic defects. This in turn could make attempts to solve social problems by improving social structures, e.g. education or employment, appear superfluous. Neglect of structural improvement in society could be the result.

As germ line genome modifications are put into practice, people might start to think that they themselves are responsible for the optimum functioning of their own genomes, as well as those of their children. In the future a human being would, after all, have access to an increasing number of genetic tests to detect potential health risks attributable to his genes. He would consequently be in a position to have them detected and thus — by adapting his lifestyle accordingly, as well as undergoing other preventive measures — reduce the risk of the disease emerging, or even stop it altogether. Should this not prove possible, he would still have the option of germ line genome modification to ensure that his offspring do not inherit the detected defect. As a result of these options some might start thinking that the outbreak of a genetically-induced disease would be the fault of either that person or his/her parents. Maybe they could have prevented the disease if only they had intervened appropriately. The outbreak of a genetic disease would therefore gradually cease to be viewed as something beyond the realm of personal responsibility, as a fateful blow; this in turn could lead to a system of rewards and sanctions within the health and insurance sectors, especially in the light of financial shortages, whereby people would be forced to undergo the relevant genetic tests and subject themselves to germ line genome modifications. Such measures would further reinforce the notion of being personally responsible for the outbreak of a genetic disease (cf. Have, 2001).

These fears cannot simply be dismissed. And yet application of germ line genome modifications in clinical practice would not automatically lead to increasing geneticization either. Maybe a growing clinical practice would encounter problems not previously envisaged, making the public aware that genetic reductionism alone is not sufficient to solve certain health issues. The enhancement of attributes with the help of corresponding germ line genome modifications might turn out to be considerably more complicated than originally thought, for example. It remains unclear, however, whether and to what extent an uncovering of such new problems would affect the notions inspired by geneticization. Moreover, a regular and critical informing of the public about the latest developments from the field of genetics would appear indicated in this context. The population at large has a far greater tendency towards reductionism with regard to genetics than the experts. This tendency could lead the public to foster unrealistic expectations concerning the potential of genetics.

Slippery slope

The slippery slope argument here refers to the problem that introducing germ line genome modifications for prevention purposes only would in time inevitably or very probably lead to the application of these techniques for the enhancement of offspring (Gardner, 1995; Krimsky, 2000; Nordgren, 2001; Winter, 2000), as well as to the morally reprehensible practice of using germ line genome modification techniques for eugenic purposes (Lunshof, 1994).

This fear is based on an assumption that, once practiced, germ line genome modifications would not be restrictable to the prevention of serious diseases, but would in time probably extend to enhancing, or even eugenic, interventions in the human germ line genome. It would be all too easy to misuse germ line genome modification techniques to enhance all sorts of genetic characteristics — starting with the correction of slight deviations from normality, and ending with the enhancement or creation of desired attributes. Since there is no clear dividing line between the pure prevention of diseases and enhancing interventions, an adequate control of germ line genome modification practices would be more or less impossible — or so the argument goes. It would only be possible if a clear definition were to be found of what constitutes a healthy person not requiring correction, and what constitutes a no longer healthy person requiring correction. And such a clear definition does not exist (cf. Juengst, 1997; Bayertz, 1991; Fletcher, 1991; Krimsky, 1990; Poliwoda, 1992; Sorg, 1992). As a result, the idea put forward by Anderson (1990), whereby clinical practice should be restricted to disease and not be permitted to include enhancement, would prove difficult to implement. This fear that, in time, gene-technological interventions could progress from the purely preventive to the enhancing should therefore be taken seriously.

Whereas eugenic developments have traditionally been driven primarily by state interests (Howel, 1991), it may be assumed that a potential eugenics of the future would be encouraged not so much from above as below. The onset of enhancing germ line genome modifications would probably be initiated by individual parents and not the state. Parents would definitely be interested in providing their future children with all the advantages available, only wanting the best for them (Capecchi, 2000; Gardner, 1995; Silver, 1997).

And yet it remains to be seen whether purely preventive germ line genome modifications really would in time lead to a practice of interventions for eugenic purposes. The development of techniques to enhance various attributes seems to have far more obstacles obstructing its path than the development of techniques to, say, prevent certain monogenetic diseases (Willgoos, 2001). It might even turn out to be completely impossible to enhance a certain attribute intentionally.

Nevertheless, the 'slippery slope' problem should not be considered closed. It is a powerful indication of the potential dangers involved in introducing germ line genome modifications without due prior deliberation, and it begs a debate on how the potential dangers in this context could be avoided.

Marginalization and exclusion of certain social groups

At a social level certain undesirable side-effects connected with the application of germ line genome modifications intended to enhance particular attributes are conceivable. Examples include the marginalization and exclusion of certain social groups. In time, the population could feel under pressure to use the available technologies to assume certain characteristics, namely those favored by society or an influential elite (Krimsky, 2000; Nordgren, 2001; Thomas, 2000). People not possessing these socially desirable characteristics — for whatever reason — would gradually become pushed to the periphery of society.

In the most likely scenario, whereby the rich have easier access to the new germ line genome modifying technologies than those less fortunate, the existing social gulf between the rich and the poor would widen further (Silver, 2000b). Two classes could emerge: the gene-technologically modified — accepted by society — and the unmodified. This would lead to a society with a discriminated lower class and a favored upper class (cf. Peters 1991).[20] Silver (1997) even

---

[20] This scenario could soon alter, however, if initially expensive technologies were to become gradually more affordable (Moore, 2000).

believes it possible that a new species of human being could emerge, crystallizing over several generations as the cumulative result of enhancing germ line genome modifications.

Be this as it may, the further exclusion of certain groups already to be found in the lower classes of society would be ethically undesirable. It would not be compatible with the notion of solidarity, not to mention its aspect of injustice (cf. Buchanan et al. 2000; Frankel & Chapman, 2000; Hughes, 2000; Parens, 2000). Since it is not at all unlikely that such a marginalization of certain social groups really would take place, this argument should be taken seriously.

Abuse of power

Another example of the undesirable long-term effects possibly resulting from germ line genome modifications intended to enhance human attributes is potential abuse of power. Enhancing germ line genome modifications could be attractive to those hungry for political power, enabling them to secure a position of dominance over others. Political power-seekers could misuse germ line genome modifications to breed people with certain attributes furthering their political cause.

This danger is relativized, however, by the fact that megalomaniacs would have far cheaper and more efficient methods at their disposal, e.g. punishment for unenvisaged copulation, forced abortion or compulsory sterilization (Birnbacher, 1994).

Reduced variety in the gene pool

Some authors believe that repeated sifting out of undesired genes would in time reduce the variety of the human gene pool. Regular germ line genome modification practice could lead to valuable genetic variations being irreversibly lost, the possession of which could have signified an evolutionary advantage for mankind in adverse circumstances — such as times of sweeping epidemics (Fukuyama, 2002; Holtug, 1997; Kitcher, 1996).

This argument is based on insecure assumptions, however (cf. Silver, 1997). It is not clear, for example, just how significant the variety of the gene pool is for the survival of the human species (Resnik et al. 1999). It is also difficult to judge the effect which germ line genome modifications would have on this genetic variety. It would probably be negligibly small if these techniques were not to be practiced *en masse* (Resnik et al. 1999).

Bearing in mind all these uncertainties, the advocates of the above argument against germ line genome modifications are called upon to give it more substance if they wish to be taken seriously. Not being able to predict what will happen — i.e. whether in the distant future it will be necessary to possess a certain gene currently known to lead to disease — is not reason enough in itself to prohibit with any conviction the application of germ line genome modification techniques — which one day might be deemed sufficiently safe (cf. Lappé, 1991). Some authors even maintain that *not* implementing germ line genome modification techniques could potentially lead to the extinction of the human race since, without the use of this technology, man may well not be sufficiently adaptable in the long term (Moseley, 1991).

7.5 Conclusion

Evaluation of the research field objectives

Here too, we shall begin by summarizing the results of the analysis with regard to the desirability of the objectives behind this research field. The first objective, the 'prevention of diseases', is extrinsically valuable. Using germ line genome modification to prevent various complaints which could not be prevented using other, less complicated means would contribute to human well-being. In addition, the burdens associated with germ line genome modifications would in some cases appear to be milder than those associated with the diseases themselves. This first objective therefore seems to be ethically desirable.

Regarding the second objective, the 'enhancement of attributes', this cannot be stated with equal conviction. There is no clear answer to the question of whether an enhancement of attributes using germ line genome modification would be fundamentally desirable or not. It is too difficult to estimate the likelihood of unfavorable circumstantial changes or certain negative effects (affecting e.g. the evolvement of other attributes) occurring. The opinions of the authors on this point diverge accordingly. Overall, the second objective does not appear to be clearly ethically desirable.

Contribution of the research field to realizing the objectives

Would germ line genome modifications really contribute to realizing the two objectives cited? The analysis reveals the following: In theory, germ line genome modifications would clearly be a method of preventing the outbreak of certain diseases, not only in treated persons but also in their offspring. The enhancement of human attributes using germ line genome modifications also appears to be at least theoretically viable. However, the technology required to realize these objectives does not actually exist yet. Its development is hindered by a number of technical obstacles which have so far proved impossible to eliminate. It therefore remains to be seen whether the prevention of diseases or the enhancement of attributes really could be realized. At present it is impossible to predict the probability of this happening. The question of whether the research field could in time contribute to a realization of these two objectives must therefore be left open.

Ethical problems

The potential problems hindering the responsible development and appropriate use of germ line genome modification techniques firstly include the risks potentially associated with them. Under certain circumstances the consequences of germ line genome modifications could be particularly negative. For example, an intended exchange of new genes for defective ones could fail, leading to severe deformities or even previously unknown genetic diseases, not only in that particular embryo, but also in the generations to come. The consequences could be devastating. And if a particular germ line genome modification technique were to require the use of manipulated viruses or bacteria, there would be a danger of new pathogens emerging which could largely devastate the human race or even destroy entire ecosystems. We can only speculate about the probability of such risks becoming reality. Maybe in the future they could be reduced to an acceptable level.

The problem of 'informed consent' is found to be a pseudo-problem. It is fundamentally impossible to obtain the consent of future generations; making it an ethical prerequisite would therefore be nonsensical. This does not mean, however, that we are absolved of all responsibility towards the generations to come.

The claim discussed in the ethical literature that germ line genome modifications are superfluous is dismissed. According to this analysis, there are some conceivable situations in which diseases could only be prevented with the help of germ line genome modifications, that is where there are no alternative or less complicated methods available — or at least not yet. As stated above, the possibility of actually using germ line genome modifications for this purpose still remains very theoretical, however.

The problems intrinsically linked with germ line genome modifications include the destruction of embryos. Here the analysis revealed the following: First of all, embryos would necessarily be destroyed in the course of numerous embryo experiments required to develop sufficiently safe technologies for the implementation of certain germ line genome modification techniques. Secondly, the preimplantation diagnostics performed within the framework of a germ line genome modification would involve the destruction of a totipotent cell, which amounts to the ethically problematic destruction of an embryo. It is conceivable however, or at least in theory, that in time diagnostic options for the detection of potential genetic defects could be developed which would not automatically involve the destruction of a totipotent cell. It is not possible to predict the likelihood of such an alternative method being developed in practice at present, however.

The problems of altered personal identity, infringement of a right to non-modified genetic material, violation of human dignity, playing God and preservation of a human genome as nature intended, all cited in the literature in connection with germ line genome modifications, were found in the analysis not to constitute insurmountable ethical problems.

Regarding the question of which undesirable effects could occur in connection with the application of germ line genome modification techniques in the longer term, the analysis produced the following results: One potential effect which cannot be dismissed is the process of geneticization which is already underway. It appears uncertain, however, whether the further development and subsequent application of germ line genome modification techniques really would spur on this undesirable process any further. The second undesirable effect potentially occurring in the longer term is the so-called 'slippery slope'. The introduction of germ line genome modifications for purely preventive purposes in time really could — due to the lack of a clear boundary between preventive and enhancing interventions — lead to the ethically reprehensible practice of using germ line genome modification techniques for eugenic purposes. It is impossible to say at present just how likely such an undesirable development would be, however. A third undesirable effect would be the exclusion of certain groups belonging to the lower social classes. This could occur as a result of using germ line genome modifications to enhance certain attributes and could favor even more the already privileged social classes. This potential effect was evaluated as needing to be taken seriously. The argument of power abuse was relativized, by contrast. Megalomaniacs could use much cheaper and more efficient methods to achieve their goals. A last undesirable effect caused by germ line genome modification could be a reduction in the variety of the gene pool. The analysis found this argument to be problematic.

Overall, the analysis revealed the following in connection with the justifiability or surmountability of the various ethical problems potentially surrounding germ line genome modifications. On the one hand, it cannot be said that all the ethical problems are justifiable or surmountable. It is, for example, unclear which tangible risks really would be involved in the further development of germ line genome modification techniques. It is also uncertain whether further development would be possible without embryo-destroying research. On the other hand — for the same reasons — it cannot be said that the ethical problems are insurmountable. The further development of *certain* germ line genome modifications which would not involve clearly unjustifiable risks or embryo-destroying research could be conceivable. The justifiability or surmountability of the ethical problems may therefore be viewed overall as problematic.

Ethical desirability

The overall result of the analysis of the research field of germ line genome modification is as follows: Of the three conditions which must be fulfilled for further development of the research field to be deemed desirable, the first is fulfilled for the first objective, preventing diseases. Its fulfillment is problematic regarding the second objective, enhancing attributes. Fulfillment of the second condition is problematic for both objectives. And the same is true of the third condition.

This means that both with regard to the objective of preventing diseases and with regard to the objective of enhancing attributes, the ethical desirability — in accordance with the criteria underlying this book — of developing germ line genome modification techniques further is questionable. The results are summarized in the following overview:

Objective	Result regarding question no.:		Condition fulfilled:		Ethical desirability
Preventing diseases	1	Objective really desirable	yes	1	Questionable
	2	Contribution uncertain	problematic	2	
	3	Surmounting of problems uncertain	problematic	3	
Enhancing attributes	1	Objective not clearly desirable	problematic	1	Questionable
	2	Contribution uncertain	problematic	2	
	3	Surmounting of problems uncertain	problematic	3	

8 INTERVENTIONS IN THE BIOLOGICAL AGING PROCESS

8.1 Research field

8.1.1 *Biogerontology*

The desire to delay old age and death, or escape from them altogether, has a long tradition (Gruman, 1966; Olshansky & Carnes, 2001). This is illustrated, for example, in the influential legends involving the eternal fountain of youth. The famous Epic of Gilgamesh, the oldest literary document stemming from the Middle East, tells the story of the powerful King Gilgamesh, who lived in Uruk in the South of Mesopotamia during the first half of the 3rd century B.C. (Sandars, 1972). In the story the King desperately attempts to elude the aging process and death. According to a tale, one could achieve eternal life by adhering to the following procedure: First of all, one needed to wash oneself with water from a particular spring. Then one had to eat a certain herb and stay awake for a whole week. Gilgamesh's attempts to fulfill these conditions fail. The King manages to find the spring and the herb; yet after he has washed himself, a snake makes off with the herb. He does not manage to stay awake for a whole week either (Sandars, 1972).

It seems as if this influential tale about the fountain of eternal youth was the origin of the negative attitude towards old age and death dominant within Western civilization. Over the course of history many attempts have been made — like Gilgamesh's — to avoid a seemingly inevitable fate. The story of Ponce de León (approx. 1460-1521), which has been handed down through the centuries, also relates a search for this fountain of eternal youth. He was a Spanish conqueror and accompanied Columbus on his second expedition (1493). In 1509 he became the first Spanish Governor of Puerto Rico. In 1512, on a search for the legendary fountain of eternal youth, he discovered the peninsula of Florida, which he began to colonize at the bidding of the King of Spain. Ponce de León unfortunately never achieved eternal life: he died from wounds he received fighting against the Native Indians (Fuson, 2000; Olshansky & Carnes, 2001).

For a long time, all sorts of quackery and fraud accompanied endeavors to overcome old age and death (Olshansky & Carnes, 2001; Olshansky et al. 2002). This was one of the reasons why serious and systematic research into the aging process did not commence until the 20th century. In the first half of the 20th century professional groups and institutions began to form, promoting investigations within the field of age research, or so-called *gerontology* (Hahn, 1992; Hayflick, 1994).[1] Following the Second World War, as a result of various successes in the areas of cellular biology, genetics and biomedicine, the development of this new field suddenly surged ahead. Influenced by knowledge and insights from these scientific fields, a new special discipline began to unfold within that of gerontology, namely *biogerontology*. Biogerontology is concerned with research into the fundamental biological processes which cause us to age. This examination of aging processes is not restricted exclusively to human beings, but also includes other organisms.

All attempts to halt the biological aging process or even reverse it have to date failed (Olshansky et al. 2002). In the 19th and 20th centuries life expectancy did dramatically increase in the Western world; yet this was primarily the consequence of a whole series of social, hygienic and medical changes and not the result of direct interventions in the aging process (Olshansky et al. 2002). This revolutionary increase in life expectancy was due to measures such as improved sewage systems, public information campaigns and the development of effective vaccinations and antibiotics (Holliday, 2000; Rose, 1999). Much more recently, however, new scientific findings from the field of biogerontology have given rise to the assumption that the biological aging process itself can be influenced and that direct interventions in this process are a viable possibility.

So far no satisfactory and complete answer has been found to the question of which concrete processes are responsible for aging and death and how they function. Various factors thought to play a role are known, but they are yet to provide a complete picture of the fundamental mechanisms underlying the aging process. Because our knowledge is still fragmentary, no technology is yet available to

---

[1] Gerontology is concerned with all aspects of aging (Ahlert, 1999). Geriatrics, by contrast, concentrates on the health problems associated with aging (Hayflick, 1994).

influence the human aging process (Olshansky et al. 2002). On the basis of the latest findings and discoveries pertaining to the biological aging process, however, several authors have already put forward initial hypotheses to this end (Bova, 1998; Clark, 1999; Fossel, 1996).

To provide a better picture of this research field, four factors thought to be involved in the aging process will first be presented, namely replicative senescence, telomeres, oxidative damage and genetics. This will be followed by a look at the proposed hypothetical ways of intervening in the human biological aging process based on these factors. Before we can begin, however, some elementary definitions must be provided. The discipline of biogerontology is still so new that many concepts have not yet become firmly established.

8.1.2 *Definitions*

Chronological and biological aging

A distinction is made between chronological aging and biological aging (Olshansky & Carnes, 2001). *Chronological* aging is understood as the growing number of years a thing exists with the passing of time (cf. Hayflick, 1994). All elements within our universe — including galaxies, stars, planets, continents, countries, books and human beings — are subject to chronological aging. The ages of all these things can — at least in theory — be determined quite precisely. The age of an element begins at the moment it first appears and steadily increases until the moment it ceases to exist.

By contrast, *biological* aging is comprehended as the process of biological changes taking place within the body of an organism over the course of time. This process of inner changes begins in an individual with conception and ends with death (cf. Hayflick, 1994; Knook, 1989). With biological aging the external symptoms — unlike the changes occurring inside the body — are easy to observe. In individuals they include things like the shortening of body height and the loss of body weight, caused by the steady deterioration of muscle and bone tissue, also increasing tiredness or waning short-term memory. The proportion of fat within the body decreases, the skin becomes wrinkled, the hair turns grey, the nails become thicker, and the head hair thins. The kidneys, lungs and pancreas function less efficiently; at a certain point in time human beings lose their ability to reproduce. Their sense of hearing, smell and taste becomes less marked. The immune system becomes weaker. Human beings become less capable of learning new things (Hayflick, 1994). Biogerontologists are attempting to discover the inner biological processes of the body which lead to these different symptoms and ultimately cause individuals to die.

The chronological and biological aging of an organism are connected insofar as that, with increasing chronological age, the biological age of an organism also advances. And yet — unlike chronological aging, which is the same for all individuals —biological aging seems to differ from person to person. Both the extent of biological aging and its actual symptoms can vary considerably, depending on the individuals in question. Taking two men, for example, one might be nearly bald at 35, whereas the other still has a full head of hair at 60. One individual might show signs of senile dementia at 65, whereas another can still be in full possession of all his mental faculties at 90.

Accidental and natural death

In connection with the causes of death, a distinction is made between death by external influence and death by internal influence. Causes of the first type of death, so-called 'accidental' death, include not having access to sufficient food, all the different types of misfortune or casualty, the various infectious diseases and all manner of violent acts. Causes of the second type of death, so-called 'natural' death, are processes taking place within the body, including the different types of cancer, hereditary diseases and cardiac arrest. Every individual who does not meet with accidental death first is eventually overtaken by natural death. The internal process of biological aging at work within every individual ultimately brings about his or her natural death. With advancing age, it also contributes to a growing risk of encountering accidental death. For example, as we get older we are increasingly at risk of contracting an infectious disease. One of the reasons for this is a gradual weakening of the body's immune system. As our locomotor system gradually deteriorates, the risk of having an accident resulting in death also increases.

Average and maximum lifespan

With regard to the duration of life, gerontologists make a distinction between 'average' and 'maximum' lifespan. The *average* lifespan of a certain group of individuals is understood as being their mean age at death. By contrast, the *maximum* lifespan of a certain species is frequently comprehended as being the mean age of the longest-living members of this species — approximately just 1% of the overall population (Clark, 1999, 14). This book employs a different, more simple definition of maximum lifespan, however, which is the greatest age which has ever been registered and well documented for one member of the species in question (Viidik, 1999). Jeanne Louise Calment (21.02.1875 [Arles] — 04.08.1997 [Arles]) attained the greatest age ever well-documented in human beings (Allard et al. 1998). The maximum lifespan for human beings is therefore said to be 122½ years.[2] It is assumed not to have changed significantly — unlike average lifespan — in the course of the past few centuries (Banks & Fossel, 1997; Olshansky & Carnes, 2001; Olshansky et al. 2002).[3] Maximum and average lifespan are partly distinguished by the fact that the former is exclusively determined by the inner biological aging process, whereas the latter is also influenced by external causes of death.

8.1.3 *Factors influencing biological aging*

Replicative senescence

The discovery of this first factor thought to play a part in the biological aging process contributed to acceptance of a new heuristic model favored by biogerontologists. This model attempts to reduce the phenomena of biological aging to processes occurring at the cellular level, or to explain them on the basis of the latter. This method was deemed worthless until well into the 1960s, primarily due to the work of well-respected French scientist Alexis Carrel (1873-1944) (Witkowski, 1980). He claimed to have kept alive a cell line of chick embryo fibroblasts over a period of more than 30 years (Carrel & Ebeling, 1921).[4] The temperature of the *in vitro* culture was maintained at that of live hens. Carrel decimated the culture regularly in order to avoid overpopulation. He also ensured that it was regularly fed with nutrients. From this experiment both Carrel and his spe-

---

[2] Expressed statistically, maximum lifespan returns a different result depending on the statistical method used. This is primarily a problem for demographers, however, and will not be addressed any further in this book.

[3] For a more precise analysis of the changes in maximum human lifespan during particular evolutionary periods, see Hofman (1984).

[4] Fibroblasts are young connective tissue cells from which connective tissue develops.

cialist colleagues concluded that individual cells themselves are immortal. Apparently they can be cultivated *in vitro* for an arbitrary period of time — or at least far beyond the maximum lifespan of a hen. They deduced that biological aging, maximum lifespan and natural death all occur only *in vivo*. They had to be caused by processes higher up than the cellular level. Carrel maintained that extracellular processes — which ultimately inflict their damaging effect on individual cells, too — were responsible for the biological aging and death of an organism (Carrel & Ebling, 1921). Carrels experiment and the conclusions he drew from it led gerontological research to concentrate for the next 40 years primarily on extracellular phenomena and processes in the search for the internal factors influencing biological aging (Witkowski, 1980). In view of the presumed immortality of individual cells there was no point, after all, in comprehending biological aging as a phenomenon at the cellular level.

In the 1960s it was discovered, however, that cells do not divide indefinitely. Instead, cells lose their division potential after a limited and definite number of divisions. In a series of skilled experiments, two young scientists, Leonard Hayflick and his colleague Paul Moorhead, were able to refute Carrel's theory (Hayflick & Moorhead, 1961; Hayflick, 1965). Hayflick established that cells *in vitro* stopped dividing after a limited and definite number of divisions. They concluded that Carrel must have made one or more errors in setting up his experiment. It was not easy for Hayflick and Moorhead to gain acceptance for their findings. Other researchers had also been unable (Shay & Wright, 2000a) to imitate Carrel's experiment and its results — keeping a cell line alive indefinitely — and yet they tended to assume that this was due to errors of their own, for example insufficient experience with this type of cell culture in the laboratory. Carrel had always emphasized that working with cell lines *in vitro* was not easy and could only be achieved with the greatest care and profound experience (Witowski, 1979). Hayflick and Moorehead refused to drop the direction their research had taken, however, and their theory was ultimately widely acknowledged by the scientific community (Clark, 1999; Hayflick, 1994; Shay & Wright, 2000a).

Hayflick and Moorehead chiefly owed this breakthrough to their convincing experimental research. One of the experiments they attempted was to bring together *in vitro* old cells harvested from a man and young cells taken from a woman. If the inability of other scientists to breed cell cultures indefinitely really had been due to a lack of skill, the result of this experiment would necessarily have been as follows: After a particular period of time, only a fraction of the original cells would still have been alive; the proportion of male to female cells would still have been more or less stable. By examining the chromosomes at the end of the allotted period, however, Hayflick and Moorehead were able to ascertain that the only cells still dividing were female cells (Hayflick & Moorhead, 1961; Hayflick, 1965 & 1994). They could more or less rule out the possibility that only male cells would suffer at the hands of erring scientists. Repeated experiments proved that this finding was not a coincidence (Hayflick, 1994).

The phenomenon whereby cells lose their division potential after a limited and definite number of divisions is known as 'replicative senescence' (Clark, 1999). This phenomenon cannot only be observed *in vitro*, but also — in all probability — *in vivo* (Faragher & Kipling, 1998). Replicative senescence is not the only way in which cells age, however. By no means all the cells within an adult organism carry on dividing until their definite end. Nevertheless, cells which by nature do not divide in adulthood still display age-related changes.[5] All cells — even those no longer dividing — tend to lose water, the older they become. This cellular dehydration causes the exterior of older organisms to change in appearance. In addition, biochemical (waste) material gathers in older cells, but is not to be found in younger cells. For example, lipofuscin — the so-called aging or 'wear and tear' pigment — collects in the intracellular granules. In very old individuals, collections of lipofuscin can cause damage to other cell bodies. They can push them away, for instance, impeding their ability to function. In time, the internal and external cell membranes become brittle, also impeding function. The composition of fluids secreted by the cells changes, also with the potential to damage anything in their immediate vicinity. One of the most important causes of cellular degeneration is oxidative damage to cell components (see below). This can affect certain proteins, but also the mitochondria or DNA of the chromosomes (Clark, 1999).

This means that even the adult cells no longer dividing display age-related changes. This may be regarded as a form of aging, and

---

[5] The model organisms instrumental to genetic research, namely the roundworm (*caenorhabditis elegans*) and the fruit-fly (*drosophila melanogaster*), have been found to have no dividing adult cells at all. And yet they also age.

may also be an internal reason for the biological aging externally perceived. Replicative senescence thus appears not to be the only type of cell aging. It cannot therefore be regarded as the only factor responsible for biological aging. Far more plausible is the hypothesis that more fundamental cellular processes exist, which in turn are responsible for the replicative senescence perceived (Clark, 1999).

Telomeres

The search for these fundamental cellular processes underlying replicative senescence raises the key issue of the factor responsible for the definite division potential of the various cell types. How do cells 'count' their divisions? Investigations have shown that so-called telomeres have the function of an internal clock (Allsop et al. 1992; Lange, 1998; Harley et al. 1990; Rhyu, 1995). Telomeres consist of long stretches of repeated DNA sequences. The sequence repeated in human beings between 1500 and 2002 times is TTAGGG. These telomeres are located at both ends of the various chromosomes. They prevent the otherwise open ends from coming into contact with other chromosomes, which would disturb both their function and their replication (Clark, 1999; Zakian, 1995).

Every time a cell divides, the telomeres lose a certain number of sequence repeats. The enzyme telomerase is capable of relengthening shortened telomeres (Allsop et al. 1995; Dahse, 1997; Greider & Blackburn, 1996; Robert, 2000; Shore, 1998), but because of the loss involved in each cell division, at some stage the moment is reached when from then on every further loss of sequence repeats can be damaging. The chromosomes could cease to be anchored in the nuclear membrane, for instance, possibly causing them to clump and, in turn, damage the DNA itself. If the damage caused by these processes reaches a critical level, after which cell-induced repair mechanisms are no longer activated, the cell in question loses its ability to divide. Cell division stops automatically when the damage ascertained at one of the various 'checkpoints' within the normal cellular cycle — where the DNA of a cell is checked for damage — is found to be no longer reparable (Dahse, 1997).

With increasing age, the ability to repair damage to genetic material, i.e. the performance of cell-induced repair mechanisms, decreases. Overall, the following cumulative effect can be observed: With increasing age, the number of cell divisions naturally increases. This means, however, that with increasing age the length of the telomeres decreases (Harley et al. 1990). As a result, DNA damage occurs more and more frequently with increasing age. Taking the decreasing ability to repair this damage, occurring with increasing age, into account as well, this could cumulatively provide an explanation for the definite division potential of a certain cell type. Consequently, telomeres appear to play a crucial role in replicative senescence (Lange, 1998; Pommier et al. 1995; Robert, 2000; Wang et al. 2000). Research findings from Bodnar et al. (1998) confirm this. In their experiments they injected an extra portion of telomerase into normal human cells and then cultivated them *in vitro*. In the part of the experiment reported in their article, the genetically modified cells survived one and a half times longer than non-modified similar cells from a control group. They showed no signs of losing their division potential either. In addition, they appeared younger with regard to their cellular morphology than the cells from the control group (Bodnar et al. 1998).

Since, however — as stated in the previous section — replicative senescence does not appear to be the only type of cell aging, its underlying mechanism, triggered by a shortening of the telomeres, cannot be regarded as the only factor responsible for the biological aging process either (Clark, 1999; Olshansky et al. 2002).[6] A hypothesis has thus been put forward that other fundamental cellular processes influencing the cellular aging of both dividing and non-dividing cells must exist (Clark, 1999).

Oxidative damage

Investigations have shown that reducing calorie intake in various animals can lengthen their lifespan (Duffy et al. 2001; Harrison & Archer, 1989; Kirk, 2001; Miller, 1999; Weindruch et al. 1986). With the help of calorie reduction it has been possible to increase not only the average lifespan of these animals, but also their maximum lifes-

---

[6] Some authors nevertheless regard telomeres as the most crucial factor determining biological aging. According to Fossel, for example, telomeres determine the maximum lifespan of an organism (Fossel, 1996). In an adult organism, not all cells divide. And yet, or so Fossel believes, the biological cellular aging of an organism can still ultimately be viewed as the result of a shortening of the telomeres in its dividing cells. Replicative senescence does not constitute an isolated phenomenon within the organism. Old cells which have exhausted their division potential could damage the functionality of non-dividing cells. Toxins could be produced, for example. Or cells could be damaged as a result of neighboring cells no longer being able to produce proteins (Fossel, 1996).

pan. Maximum lifespan might not be an absolute parameter anyway, as clearly shown in experiments conducted by McCay et al. back in the 1930s (McCay et al. 1935; McCay et al. 1939). McCay investigated in rats the connection between their maximum lifespan and the speed with which they achieved their full physical growth. He attempted to induce a longer lifespan in a certain rat population by delaying their development to full growth. This delayed growth was achieved in the designated rat population by administering it fewer calories. The rats received less food than normal, albeit enriched with extra vitamins and minerals. A control group was allowed to satisfy its hunger *ad libitum*. The 'diet rats' proved to be extraordinarily healthy. Both their average and their maximum lifespan increased by 50 to 80%. Later experiments confirmed the most important findings from McCay's experiments.

More recent research has suggested, however, that delayed physical growth as such is not responsible for this effect on lifespan (Clark, 1999). A prolonged lifespan can also be clearly registered in already fully grown animals which are then subjected to a reduced calorie intake. Consequently, it is not the delay in growth which constitutes the most important factor in achieving a longer lifespan, but a reduction in calorie intake. The results of these experiments and how they should be interpreted are still being debated, however. Some authors maintain that the laboratory animals used as a control group, permitted to eat *ad libitum*, should be regarded as abnormal. In the outside world they would have more exercise and find less food. Quite possibly, the animals in the control group shortened their lifespan by overeating. Following this interpretation, the maximum lifespan in these animals was shortened, and not *vice versa* (Olshansky et al. 2002).

In the search for an explanation regarding the effect on lifespan of reducing calorie intake, oxidative damage has been found to play an important role (Clark, 1999; Weindruch, 1996). When oxygen and hydrogen react in the mitochondria to form water, so-called oxygen radicals result. These intermediates of the oxidation process can behave very reactively. Normally they remain in the mitochondria, where they are converted to H_2O. But they can also escape and cause damage as so-called 'free' oxygen radicals to cellular molecules, such as proteins or lipids. In addition, they can damage the DNA in the mitochondria themselves, which can lead to disturbances in the energy household, and in turn impede crucial cell functions (Miquel

& Fleming, 1986).[7] Oxygen radicals can permeate damaged mitochondria more easily. The intermediates of the oxidation reaction can thus cause substantial damage, both inside the mitochondria and outside them — when they escape (Weindruch, 1996). This cell damage caused by oxygen radicals is known as 'oxidative damage'. Oxidative damage to protein molecules can disturb important enzyme functions, for example. Oxidized lipids can contribute to the development of arteriosclerosis. The DNA of the cell nucleus can also suffer severe oxidative damage. If this damage becomes sufficiently great — as already mentioned above — the cells lose their potential to divide. Division stops automatically when the damaged is registered by one of the 'checkpoints' within the cellular cycle. As oxidative damage increases, so does the risk of developing diseases like cancer or cardiovascular complaints (Clark, 1999).

Over the course of evolution, organisms have developed various mechanisms to counteract oxidative damage. In the human body, for example, hemoglobin alone transports oxygen to the cells, preventing it from causing damage to any other components within the blood. Special antioxidizing enzymes, such as catalase, eliminate free oxygen radicals. And there are various repair mechanisms in the body responsible for restoring or eliminating damaged lipids and proteins. Corresponding repair mechanisms have developed especially to deal with the oxidative damage caused to DNA — which appears to play such an important role in the biological aging process. With increasing age the performance of these mechanisms and thus the body's ability to repair the damage, deteriorates. The following cumulative effect results: The number of free oxygen radicals increases with the intake of calories. Their ability to cause oxidative damage also increases, meaning that with increasing calorie intake more and more oxidative damage is inflicted on the cells. At the same time, the ability to repair or eliminate this damage decreases with age. The net effect of oxidative damage thus increases with age, meaning that this process could play a role in explaining cellular, and ultimately biological, aging (Clark, 1999).

This hypothesis regarding the role of oxidative damage could explain the prolonged lifespan in selected animals administered with fewer calories. After all, the perpetrators of the damage — the oxy-

---

[7] The extent to which such damage to the mt-DNA influences the biological aging of human beings is still being debated, however (Grey, 2000).

gen radicals — are released when calories are burnt to produce energy. If calorie intake is minimized, only a minimum of free oxygen radicals can be released. The resulting oxidative damage is then less, reducing the risk of certain idiopathic diseases and possibly even delaying the biological aging process (Clark, 1999).

The genetic connection

Biogerontological research is also concerned with the genetic involvement in biological aging (Jazwinski, 1996; Zant & Haan, 1999). No special genetic programs are required for the biological aging process (Hayflick, 2000; Kirkwood, 1996 & 1999; Miller, 1999; Olshansky & Carnes, 2001; Olshansky et al. 2002), but this does not render genes fundamentally irrelevant to it (Miller, 1999; Rattan, 1998). In the literature there has already been extensive discussion about the significance of particular genes for the process of biological aging (Zant & Haan, 1999). A uniform terminology for these genes is still wanting, however. Some speak of *gerontogenes* (Johnson et al. 1996 & 2000; Rattan, 1995, 1998 & 2000a), and this is the term also favored in this book, others of *longevity assurance genes* (Jazwinski, 1996).

To date various genes thought to be particular significant with regard to longevity or aging have been investigated, including in yeast (*saccharomyces cerevisiae*) (D'mello et al. 1994; Guarente, 1997; Jazwinski, 1996; Jazwinski, 1998; Jazwinski, 1999; Sinclair et al. 1997), in roundworms (*caenorhabditis elegans*) (Guarente, 1997; Jazwinski, 1996; Jazwinski, 1998; Johnson et al. 2000 & 2001; Kimura et al. 1997; Lakowski & Hekimi, 1996; Lin et al. 1997; Morris et al. 1996; Ogg et al. 1997), in fruit-flies (*drosophila melanogaster*) (Lin et al. 1998) and in mammals (Gelman et al. 1988; Jazwinski, 1996; Migliaccio et al. 1999; Miller et al. 1998; Haan et al. 1998). In human beings various genetic structures thought to be connected with longevity have also been discovered (Jazwinski, 1996; Jian-Gang et al. 1998; Schächter et al. 1994).

Some of the so-called gerontogenes might contain codes for maintenance or repair mechanisms (Clark, 1999). These mechanisms could include protection from oxidative damage, DNA repairs or safe ways of transferring genetic information (Holliday, 2000). The sheer variety of genes which have so far been connected with aging or longevity indicates that the various species, in addition to the genes they have in common — containing codes for maintenance or repair mechanisms, for example — maybe also possess genetic structures unique to their species, containing codes for their own gerontogenetic mechanisms (Rattan, 2001).

Evolutionary theories also lead us to suppose that aging genes have not developed in order to cause aging and establish a maximum lifespan (Kirkwood & Austad, 2000). The biogerontologist Suresh Rattan, for example, believes that the registered 'genetic regulation' of lifespan should be comprehended as an indirect effect of the genetic coding determining a so-called *essential lifespan*. He understands an 'essential lifespan' as being the period of time required for successful reproduction and guaranteed survival of the next generation (Rattan 2000a, 2000b & 2001). 'Genetic regulation' should thus be viewed less as a direct control of aging, and more as an indirect influencing of the same (Hayflick, 1994; Olshansky et al. 2002). The aging phenomenon does not seem to be so much evolutionary intention as far more the consequence of evolutionary neglect (Carnes et al. 1999; Faragher & Kipling, 1998; Olshansky et al. 2001 & 2002; Rattan, 1998; Rose, 1999 & 2000; Wick et al. 2000).

8.1.4 *Possible interventions in the biological aging process*

Could it really be possible to delay the biological aging process and maybe even to prolong the maximum human lifespan using certain controlled interventions? The most important prerequisite before we can answer this question seriously would be sufficient knowledge of all, or at least the most crucial, factors triggering biological aging. Only then can possible interventions be soundly investigated. To date, however, our understanding of biological aging most probably does not include all the contributing factors (Ahlert, 1999; Cristofalo, 1991; McClearn, 1997). For this reason, any presentation of possible interventions must remain fundamentally speculative.

Nevertheless, the current findings of biogerontological research pertaining to the foundations of biological aging have given various authors cause enough to speculate about possible ways of intervening in this process. In particular the biogerontological research findings regarding telomeres, oxidative damage and the genetic foundation of aging have served as sources of inspiration. It should once again be emphasized, however, that these are only hypotheses. Numerous publications are already in print which contain detailed treatments or methods to delay, halt or even reverse the aging process (Carper, 1996; Chopra, 2001; Klatz & Kahn, 1998; Pierpaoli et al. 1995), and yet not one of the ideas in these works has been scientifically verified (Austad, 1997; Banks & Fossel, 1997; Holliday, 2000; Olshansky et al. 2002).

According to Michael Fossel (1996), it is the telomeres which are especially responsible for biological aging. In his view, they cause so-called replicative senescence, which in turn contributes to biological aging. On the basis of this hypothesis, Fossel believes an intervention in the biological aging process based on the enzyme telomerase to be a viable possibility (cf. Glannon, 2002a & 2002b). This enzyme could relengthen shortened telomeres, thus counteracting replicative senescence. Although every cell has telomerase genes, in most cells these genes are not expressed. In many fully-grown somatic cells the enzyme is not to be found at all. It would thus seem an obvious step to develop a method which would enable telomerase to be introduced to these cells. The enzyme could then relengthen the telomeres in the cells and indirectly extend the latter's division potential, in turn delaying the biological aging process.

There would still be the difficulty, however, of how to introduce the enzyme. A simple injection would fail because enzymes in the blood would rapidly destroy the telomerase enzyme. Fossel proposes three solutions to this problem. The first consists in injecting not the original telomerase liable to destruction, but an artificially produced, more robust variety. This 'ersatz telomerase' could be constructed by performing minor chemical modifications to the original molecule, enabling it to retain its function for hours or even days (Fossel, 1996).

Fossel continues with his second possibility, which presupposes knowledge of the exact DNA sequence of the genes coding for telomerase. Assuming this knowledge, the sequence could be copied *in vitro* and the genes thus produced then introduced to the target cells. This introduction would be performed with the help of liposomes or viral vectors. Fossel believes this second possibility to be somewhat problematic, however. For example, the exact cells requiring a genetic intervention would be difficult to recognize. And why should artificially introduced genes express themselves if natural ones do not? How could the activity of the 'artificial' genes be controlled? Uncontrolled and indefinite telomerase production could result in gigantic telomeres, potentially leading to all sorts of complications. For example, they could increase the risk of cancer (Fossel, 1996).

Fossel's third option is directed at the telomerase genes which are to be found in all cells, but which are normally inactive. Possibly they could be activated with a kind of 'telomerase driver'. A biochemical compound would have to be developed which could stimulate the telomerase genes to become active. Via the dosage and effectiveness of the compound, as well as the rapidity with which it could be destroyed again, the amount of telomerase produced and the extent of telomere growth could be controlled (Fossel, 1996).

Not only telomeres, but also research into the role played in the biological aging process by oxidative damage has inspired thoughts about interventions in this process. Since there is a direct link between oxidative damage and the burning of foodstuffs, it should in principle be possible to combat the aging process by restricting one's calorie intake. Whole series of animal experiments confirm this theory. The potential effects on human biological aging of reducing calorie intake have yet to undergo systematic investigation, and yet various authors believe that there is no reason to assume that reduced calorie intake would *not* delay the biological aging process in human beings (Arking, 1998; Clark, 1999; Lane et al. 2002).

In addition to calorie reduction there are also other conceivable ways of intervening in the biological aging process — on the basis of the hypothesis that oxidative damage is partly responsible for biological aging. They might include genetic interventions aimed specifically at those genes containing coding for antioxidative enzymes, such as catalase. Also possible would be the introduction of additional genes coding for hunger-suppressing proteins, such as leptin (Clark, 1999, 217; Weindruch, 1996). Of the antioxidative supplements already on the market, not one has so far been scientifically proven to have an actual influence on human biological aging (Olshansky et al. 2002).[8]

Finally — as mentioned above — the hypothesis has been put forward that biological aging might be at least partly and indirectly influenced by genetic factors. If this genetic connection with regard to biological aging were to become known, it might be possible to perform a genetic intervention in human beings to prolong their lifespan (Chadwick, 1999; Rose, 1999; Vijg, 1990). This has already been achieved in other species. Various authors believe it improbable, however, that biological aging could be influenced in a controlled manner using genetic interventions. In all probability there are no

---

[8] In fruit-flies and roundworms a positive link between the concentration of antioxidative enzymes and maximum lifespan has been observed. This link has not been established in warm-blooded animals, however (Grey, 2000).

genes which directly control the aging process (Olshansky et al. 2002; Rattan, 1997 & 1998).

8.2 Evaluation of the research field objectives

8.2.1 *Objectives*

Increasing the preventive and therapeutic options available

The primary hopes attached to research into biological aging for the purpose of developing ways of influencing it are improved prevention and therapy of diseases connected with aging (Banks & Fossel, 1997; Glannon, 2002a & 2002b; Holliday, 2000; Knook, 1989; Miller, 1997; Olshansky et al. 2002; Vijg, 1990; Wick et al. 2000). These diseases include osteoarthritis, cancer, cardiovascular diseases and dementia (Robert, 2000; Wick et al. 2000). Further development in this research field also promises a better understanding of the syndromes collectively known as 'progeria'. Patients with these syndromes — such as the Hutchinson-Gilford, Werner's or the Hallerman-Streiff-François syndrome — display symptoms of premature aging at an abnormally young age (Clark, 1999).[9]

Extending the maximum lifespan

A further objective behind interventions in the biological aging process is to extend the maximum lifespan (Banks & Fossel, 1997; Clark, 1999; Fossel, 1996; Vijg, 1990). In the future, selected interventions could possibly manipulate the normal biological aging process in order to delay it. In time this could lead to an increase in maximum age. As a result, human beings would have — at least in theory — quantitatively more lifetime at their disposal than ever before.

8.2.2 *Evaluation*

Increasing the preventive and therapeutic options available

At first sight any improvement in the treatment of diseases is fundamentally desirable, therefore including that of age-related diseases.

---

[9] Incidentally, biogerontologists find it difficult to make a precise terminological distinction between natural biological aging as a *physiological* process and the diseases associated with natural biological aging as a *pathological* process (Holliday, 2000). Bearing in mind the objectives analyzed here, it would appear necessary that biogerontologists make an effort to introduce more clarity in this respect.

This is only really true, however, if the latter really can be prevented, cured or at least symptomatically treated by intervening in the biological aging process. If only a patient's life expectancy were to be altered as a result of such interventions, and not the course of his disease, a longer life would quite possibly merely prolong his suffering, which would not be clearly desirable.

Since all effective therapies can improve patient health or — failing that — at least help to alleviate suffering, they are held in high esteem. Effective prevention can hinder a particular disease from developing and thus nip in the bud any associated suffering. Both the prevention of age-related diseases and the discovery of new ways of treating them could thus contribute to the health and well-being of mankind — two more highly esteemed phenomena. Prevention and treatment of age-related diseases may thus be regarded as extrinsically valuable.

This objective can therefore be evaluated as actually desirable. This is especially true in view of the fact that mankind is growing steadily older. Many current forms of geriatric therapy are still oriented to the effects of aging, but not to their cause, the aging process itself. A better understanding of the biological aging process, as well as of methods to influence this process, could prove helpful in this respect (Olshansky et al. 2002).

In the case of progeria — which might perhaps be comprehended as a pathological variation of biological aging (Clark, 1999) — a development of preventive options, as well as an increase in therapeutic options, would appear to be particularly desirable. This would prevent not only unnecessary suffering, but also premature death, a regular occurrence in patients with progeric diseases. Life is the prerequisite for all other worthy experiences (cf. Callahan, 1998). If a person is robbed of it prematurely, a fulfilled existence is often thwarted (cf. Callahan, 1987). Premature deaths in cases such as these are generally also experienced as tragic.

Extending the maximum lifespan

At first sight, this objective — extending the maximum lifespan and theoretically granting man more time to live — also appears to be desirable. Two considerations relativize this *prima facie* positive evaluation, however. The first questions the motives behind this objective. Why should man desire to prolong his maximum lifespan? Is it really a problem that human beings cannot become much older than 120? If so, this problem cannot be connected with the pace of normal human biological aging. Disregarding those who die a natural or accidental death not related to biological aging (e.g. through Huntington's disease or a tragic traffic accident), people aging at normal speed can now become 80, 90 or 100, maybe even 120. This is a length of time generally providing enough scope for a fulfilled life (cf. Callahan, 1987 & 1990). Why wish to extend it further? What desires are buried within this wish?

It may well be less the circumstance that man can only become 80 to 120 years old, and far more the fact that his life ends at all, which is the real reason behind this wish to prolong the human lifespan. The inevitable way of things always was, and still is, a frequent source of uneasiness and fear. Throughout the ages, attempts have been made to delay or escape old age and death, even documented in the earliest literary works known to man (see 8.1.1). The reason for this disquiet and anxiety possibly lies in the complex quest to grasp the meaning of life — particularly in view of the transience of all things. What is the point of all man's efforts when ultimately everything — even he — fades away? The 'meaning of life in the light of human mortality' puzzle is not suddenly going to be solved by slowing down the biological aging process to prolong the end, however. This would not render man immortal, but merely enable him to die later. An attempt to duck out of a confrontation with such a fundamental issue as the meaning of life constitutes a strategy of avoidance which cannot be regarded as positive.

The second consideration concerns the potentially negative effects that longevity could have on the quality of human life. Quantity of life and quality of life do not necessarily go hand-in-hand, as illustrated long ago in the Greek legend of Tithonus. This Trojan prince was one of several handsome mortals to be stolen away by Eos, the goddess of the dawn. Eos took Tithonus to Ethiopia, where she bore him two sons, Emathion and Memnon. According to legend, Eos managed to persuade Zeus to grant Tithonus immortality. She forgot to ask for eternal youth as well, though, and was forced to watch as Tithonus gradually became older and wizened (Bulfinch, 1998).

In the field of medicine we have also been able to observe an increasing discrepancy between quantity of life and quality of life. The rapid development of medical technology over the past few decades has made it possible to keep people alive at even the most basic of levels of existence and under the most wretched of circumstances. The quality of life prevailing in such situations often seems to be unbearably low. As a result of this development, the goal of preserving life whatever the circumstances is no longer generally accepted or striven for. The view now exists that not only the duration of life, but also its quality, should be taken into account when technology is to be used to keep patients alive. Many physicians now accept, for example, that medication to relieve pain and other unpleasant symptoms may even be administered if it will probably shorten a patient's life. In this case quality of life carries more weight than quantity of life.

But how would an intervention to delay the normal biological aging process affect the quality of human life? It should, at the very least, not be taken for granted that such a delay would automatically increase our quality of life (cf. Baltes, 1999; Kirkwood, 1996). Quality of life is influenced by physical, psychological, social and spiritual factors. It is conceivable that interventions to delay a person's biological aging might lead to feelings of isolation, alienation and loneliness. Problems such as these are already occurring amongst the elderly in modern industrial societies. Mass interventions to delay the biological aging process could well intensify the problem (McKeefery, 1981). It is also conceivable that certain diseases would seek out a far greater number of people, likewise having a negative effect on their quality of life. We do not yet know the true long-term effects of delaying the biological aging process, and yet if such interventions were ever to become freely available in the future, a critical examination of their effects on quality of life would be indicated.

In summary, the normal human lifespan as we know it today facilitates a fulfilled life. The reason for wanting longevity is therefore not in order to be able to look back later on a full life. Far more, motives of repression and strategies of avoidance seem to be involved. The puzzle that is the meaning of life in the light of the transience of all human activities, as well as the vanity of all human ambitions, would not be solved by delaying the end of life, however. Coping with mortality does not suddenly become any easier by putting up the maximum age limit. Because we have so little knowledge about it to date, the potential consequences of delaying the normal biological aging process are unclear. It is thus currently impossible to say what effect delaying normal aging would have on human well-being. This means that a clearly positive evaluation of this objective is not possible at the present time.

8.3 Contribution of the research field to realizing the objectives

8.3.1 Increasing the preventive and therapeutic options available

To date, no methods or interventions are known which have been proven to influence the biological aging process (Austad, 1997; Olshansky et al. 2002). And, as has already been mentioned, at this stage of biogerontological research the possible approaches to intervening in this process are all still extremely hypothetical and speculative. It remains to be seen whether they will ever be realized. Maybe, as knowledge about the factors influencing biological aging grows, completely new and previously unknown possibilities will unfold. A potential discovery that controlled and specifically directed interventions in the biological aging process are fundamentally impossible cannot be ruled out either.

A basic prerequisite would be the possession of a viable theory about human biological aging. A uniform and generally accepted theory explaining biological aging in an integral manner does not yet exist, however (Ahlert, 1999; Cristofalo, 1991; McClearn, 1997). We do not even have a generally accepted definition of aging (Hayflick, 1994; Miller, 1999; Robert, 1999 & 2000). Instead, numerous different theoretical approaches attempt to explain it (Kirkwood, 1998; McClearn, 1997; Medvedev, 1990). We would be justified in doubting whether a complete and uniform theory on biological aging could ever be developed. Various authors are currently of the opinion that aging is a multi-dimensional, multi-causal and stochastic process (Hayflick, 2000; Takahashi, 2000; Rattan, 1998 & 2001). Rattan (2001), for example, believes the wide variety of phenotypical aging phenomena to be an indication of the fact that biological aging includes different processes at different levels. Firstly, aging processes vary from one species to another; secondly, they vary within one species from individual to individual; thirdly they vary within one individual from organ to organ and tissue type to tissue type; fourthly, they vary within one organ from cell to cell; and finally, they vary within one cell from macromolecule to macromolecule (Rattan, 2001).

There may not yet exist an integral and generally accepted theory of biological aging, but maybe the growth in biogerontological knowledge expected in the near future will open up some new prospects. It is at least theoretically conceivable that in time controlled interventions in the biological aging process might become feasible (Olshansky et al. 2002). This would mean that increasing the preventive and therapeutic options available in conjunction with aging would enter the realms of possibility. It remains to be seen whether this could really be achieved by intervening in the biological aging process, however.

8.3.2 *Extending the maximum lifespan*

For the same reasons as above (see 8.3.1) it appears to be fundamentally uncertain whether man will ever be capable of extending his maximum lifespan by controlled intervention in his own biological aging process. The development of such interventions cannot be ruled out, however, at least theoretically (Arking, 1998; Banks & Fossel, 1997; Clark, 1999; Fossel, 1996; Rose, 1999; Rose & Nusbaum, 1994; Vijg, 1990). After all, the maximum lifespans of certain animal species have already been successfully extended using different methods (cf. Banks & Fossel, 1997). As described in 8.1.3, McCay was able to achieve an extension of the maximum lifespan in rats by reducing their calorie intake. Genetic interventions have led to similar results in roundworms (Lakowski & Hekimi, 1996) and fruit-flies (Orr & Sohal, 1996; Clark, 1999). How exactly these experiments should be interpreted, however, is still being debated. It is apparently still unclear whether these experiments really did involve interventions to delay the biological aging process and thus to extend the maximum lifespans of these animals (Olshansky et al. 2002).

If we assume for a moment that these experiments really did manage to delay biological aging in the animals used, then — at least in theory — similar interventions could be possible in human beings. It is impossible to know whether such interventions would ever be practicable, however, and a prognosis regarding the probability of this happening is likewise out of the question.

8.4 Ethical problems

8.4.1 *Problems of responsible development and appropriate use*

Risks

To date, no methods of influencing the biological aging process are available (Austad, 1997; Olshansky et al. 2002). As a logical result of this, the risks potentially connected with interventions in the biological aging process can only be presented hypothetically, with no factual foundation. A real scenario, involving not only the exact way in which such an intervention may be conducted, but also relevant experiments leading up to its development, is lacking. The author of this study has also failed to find any appropriate and earnest scenarios in the biogerontological literature. One such scenario would be necessary for any well-founded postulations on this topic, however. Substantiated reflection on the risks involved therefore does not seem to be possible at the current stage of biogerontological investigation. We will just have to await the development of actual human experiments.

Should it become possible to conduct such experiments, however, each individual experiment would immediately and separately have to be evaluated for its potential risks. The first step would be to examine the research protocols, necessarily drawn up in the course of developing such interventions. If the risks were still to remain largely unknown after this examination, then for the sake of a sound risk assessment human experiments would have to be temporarily forfeited in favor of experiments conducted exclusively using appropriate animal models. If it should still prove impossible to produce a substantiated risk assessment, there would of course be no ethical justification for human experiments. The proportionality of an experiment needs to be estimated positively — i.e. the risks and burdens of the experiment on the one hand, together with its possible advantages on the other hand, must be in a ratio deemed acceptable — before it can be conducted in an ethically non-reprehensible manner.

8.4.2 Problems intrinsically linked with the technology

The goals of medicine

In the 1990s, the Hastings Center, a U.S. Center for Medical Ethics in New York State, initiated a project entitled *The Goals of Medicine* to research the current aims of the medical world (HC, 1996). In the light of 20th century economic, social and scientific developments, the Center wanted to investigate whether traditional medical goals needed updating. Using selected consensus procedures, a critical survey of goals was conducted in fourteen countries. According to the results of this international investigational project, the following four points were found to be the goals of medicine:

(1) Disease and injury prevention, as well as the promotion and maintenance of health;
(2) Alleviation of pain and suffering caused by disease;
(3) Care for, and healing of, the sick, as well as care for the incurably sick;
(4) Avoidance of premature death, as well as aspiration towards peaceful death.

In our analysis of the ethical problems intrinsically linked with interventions to delay the biological aging process, the following question now arises: Would the purpose behind interventions aimed at extending the maximum lifespan be included in any of these four goals? In order to answer this question, each individual goal will be viewed separately.

Goal 1 (Disease and injury prevention, as well as the promotion and maintenance of health): The extent to which delaying normal biological aging could be assigned to this first goal depends on the relationship perceived between the normal biological aging process and the phenomena of disease and health. This perception is in turn based on the favored conceptions of disease and health.

With regard to health, *positive* and *negative* conceptions can be distinguished. The *negative* conception of health describes it in terms of what it is not: Health is the absence of disease. A person is healthy if he is not sick. This conception is widespread amongst the population at large. On the basis of this definition, disease and injury prevention are identical to the maintenance of health. The only way of maintaining health is to prevent disease and injury. Following this view, promotion of health is not possible. If somebody is healthy — i.e. not sick or injured — his condition cannot be raised any higher.

Taking this definition of health, would delaying the biological aging process fall under the first goal? This would only be the case if one were to regard the normal biological aging process as a disease. Is that permissible? And if so, to what degree? Our first intuition is not to regard aging as a disease (cf. Glannon, 2002a; Hayflick, 2000; Reznek, 1987). Otherwise life itself would already imply disease in its inextricable links to the aging process. This in turn would stretch the concept of disease to such limits that it could no longer be used reasonably.[10] On the basis of this negative definition of health, delaying

---

[10] Nevertheless, there is much discussion about whether biological aging should be regarded as a disease (Caplan, 1992; Chadwick, 1999).

the normal biological aging process therefore cannot be included within the first goal.

The *positive* conception of health attributes more constituents to this state than the mere non-existence of disease (Have et al. 1998). Various sub-conceptions, each attributing different additional elements to health, can be distinguished: The *biological* view, for example, comprehends health as being the ideal adaptation of the body to its environment. The more the body can do this, the healthier it is. The *statistical* view of health sees it as the physical and mental human state most frequently occurring within a society. For the *psychological* view of health, the extent of self-fulfillment or inner harmony plays an important role. The *sociological* definition of health concentrates on the degree to which an individual is able to function within society. The better the individual functions, the healthier he is regarded as being. And following the *political* view — the definition used, incidentally, by the World Health Organization — health is a state of complete physical, mental and social well-being (Have et al. 1998).

Could delaying the normal biological aging process therefore be counted as belonging to the first goal if a *positive* definition of health is assumed? Taking the political definition of health, interventions to delay the normal biological aging process could be viewed as health-promoting, provided that these interventions really did contribute to physical, mental and social well-being. However, working with this political view of health in combination with the semi-goal of promoting and maintaining health appears to be problematic. It would potentially mean that the responsibility for achieving and maintaining this state of complete physical, mental and social well-being in the citizens of a state would be shouldered by the health sector. And this, in turn, would not only mean unreasonable demands on medical responsibility; it would also mean that, in time, the number of activities occupying the health sector would grow beyond control, since striving towards complete well-being would justify all manner of steps. The boundaries of the health sector would start to blur, and the door would be opened to unrestricted medicalization — quite apart from the fact that the health sector could never realize the envisaged goal anyway. A political definition of health would therefore not really be practicable. For this reason it seems irrelevant that, according to this view, delaying the normal biological aging process could possibly be included within the first goal.

Taking the various psychological definitions of health — comprehending it as meaning a state of complete contentment or perfect happiness, for example — the consequences would be similar to those described above. And the same is true for sociological definitions — perceiving health as a state of total integration in a society, for example. These two viewpoints therefore also have to be discounted from our analysis of whether delaying the normal biological aging process can be included within the first goal on the basis of a *positive* definition of health.

The statistical viewpoint described health as being the physical and mental state occurring most frequently within a society. In this case, delaying the normal biological aging process would be pointless. Only extremely accelerated aging would count as a state requiring medical treatment. Normal biological aging would, after all, represent the most frequently occurring phenomenon within society.

And finally the biological view — defining health as the ideal adaptation of a body to its environment — would not enable interventions to delay the normal biological aging process to be seen as health-maintaining or health-promoting. Delaying the biological aging process would have no influence on the degree of adaptation of an organism to its environment.

Overall, then, we can establish that the delaying of the normal biological aging process, envisaged with the help of appropriate interventions, would not fall under the first goal — disease and injury prevention, as well as the promotion and maintenance of health. This seems to be very clear based on the negative conception of health. On the basis of the positive conception, delaying the normal biological aging process could not be seen as health-promoting or health-maintaining taking the statistical or biological definitions of health. Assignment to this first goal would not be out of the question taking the political, psychological or sociological definitions, but these conceptions of health would entail such grave disadvantages that proceeding down any of these paths would not seem a good idea.

Goal 2 (Alleviation of pain and suffering caused by disease): It is not possible to include a delay of the normal biological aging process within this goal of medicine. Merely delaying old age does not alleviate any pain or suffering caused by disease.

Goal 3 (Care for, and healing of, the sick, as well as care for the incurably sick): Delaying the normal biological aging process could not be assigned to this goal of medicine either. Human beings subject to the normal biological aging process cannot be regarded as sick. We can therefore not speak of caring for or healing the sick, and certainly not of caring for the incurably sick in the context of these interventions.

Goal 4 (Avoidance of premature death, as well as aspiration towards peaceful death): Whether delaying the normal biological aging process could be included within this last goal of medicine depends on the more fundamental question of whether such interventions could facilitate the avoidance of premature death at all. To investigate this, we shall distinguish three different types of death.

The first type comprises *natural deaths which are not attributable to the normal biological aging process*, for example due to hereditary diseases such as Huntington's disease. These deaths can occur prematurely, i.e. before the sufferer has been able to live a 'fulfilled life'.[11] Interventions to delay the aging process have no influence on this first type of natural death.

The second type comprises *natural deaths which are attributable to the normal biological aging process*, commonly referred to as 'death through old age'. These deaths occur relatively late, however. It is generally opined that a death between the ages of 70 and 100 — the normal range for most natural deaths of this second type — is not an obstacle to realizing a fulfilled life. If this second type of natural death is not deemed to be 'premature', however, then a measure to avoid premature death in this context would be nonsensical.

The third type of death viewed here comprises *accidental deaths*, i.e. deaths caused by external influences.[12] The probability of dying an accidental death increases with biological age, a process taking place within every individual. This probability does not rise sharply, however, until an age of somewhere between 50 and 70. Some deaths

---

[11] Views vary enormously regarding what constitutes a fulfilled life. Generally speaking, the term 'premature death' is often used to refer to somebody who dies at a young age — for example a man at the beginning of his career, who leaves behind a young wife and small children.

[12] Examples of this third type include all manner of misadventure and casualty, as well as the various infectious diseases.

within this last category can certainly be deemed 'premature'. The possibility of avoiding them by delaying the normal biological aging process could thus be a matter for discussion. Such interventions might actually be able to reduce the risk of premature accidental death.

Conclusion: Overall — apart from the abovementioned premature accidental deaths which could be a matter for discussion — delaying the normal biological aging process cannot then be said to fall within any of the four goals with which, according to the results of the Hastings Center's *The Goals of Medicine* project, the field of medicine should be occupying itself.

One objection to this conclusion could be that whilst delaying the normal biological aging process might not count as one of the cited goals of modern medicine, it certainly is in accord with a very traditional goal, the preservation of life, which dates back to Hippocrates. The following two points can be made at this juncture: Firstly, in retrospect, this traditional goal was valuable within the context of a medicine capable of little else other than the alleviation of symptoms. Thus seen, the preservation of life has constituted an important norm throughout the history of medicine. The rapid medical developments over the last century — and particularly the last decades — have meant an explosion in the medical options available, however. The present medical possibilities permit life to be preserved even when it is barely reasonable. In order to facilitate the circumvention of such a situation, and not to have to preserve life at all costs, there has recently been a conscious departure from this traditional goal (HC, 1996).
    Secondly, digging out a former goal of medicine in order to evaluate the purpose of a medical intervention which will not be conducted until some time into the future — and maybe never — seems somewhat anachronistic. At the time when this traditional goal of preserving life was deemed appropriate, nobody thought it possible that one day life could be prolonged by intervening in the biological aging process, let alone considered this possibility when formulating the goal.

Personal identity

The bioethicist Walter Glannon (2002b) believes that significantly prolonging life would involve an undesirable alteration to personal identity. In his opinion, the links between a human being's various consecutive states of consciousness would weaken with time, depending on the extent of the longevity. After a certain period of time the same body would encase a new person. If a human being were to live for long enough — were the lifespan of his body to be sufficiently prolonged — a whole series of different people could succeed each other within it. The body would then merely serve as a basis for the various biographies of these different people.

Glannon illustrates his point with a reference to the life of Methuselah, a figure from the Bible (Gen 5,21ff).[13] When Methuselah reached the age of 100, he could still remember his early childhood. At the age of 150 he could only remember events he had witnessed after his 20th year. By the age of 200 he only had memories from his 70s onwards. And on his 969th birthday — in the year that he died (Gen 5,27) — Methuselah could hardly remember anything from before his 839th year. Similar things happened with Methuselah's views or opinions and personality. By his 220th year, both had changed completely from what they had been at the age of 90.

Assessing Methuselah's development, Glannon puts forward the following two theses: (1) Over its lifespan of nearly 1000 years, Methuselah's body housed several different people. His personal identity altered on several occasions. (2) It would not have been rational for the young Methuselah to want to have anything to do with the old Methuselah. The two of them, the young and the old Methuselahs, were completely different people. On the basis of these two theses, Glannon draws the following conclusion: A long life such as that lived by Methuselah is not desirable. Glannon extends this evaluation to include not just 'Methuselahean' lifespans but every significant prolonging of human life. For him a longevity of just 200 years already ceases to be desirable (Glannon, 2002b).

The central issue here, of whether personal identity really would alter during a significantly prolonged human lifespan, hinges on the criterion selected to determine personal identity. Criteria for personal identity can be divided into two categories. The first group includes criteria based on physical attributes conveying personal identity; the second group includes those based on psychological attributes.[14]

---

[13] Glannon borrows this example from Lewis (1976).

[14] Discussion still continues as to which criterion is the best yardstick for personal identity (Gordijn, 1996).

Glannon clearly presumes a criterion from the second category in his analysis. For him the continuity of Methuselah's body is irrelevant, for example. If we *were* to take continuity of the body as the criterion for personal identity, Methuselah's long lifespan would prove no problem as far as his personal identity was concerned — presuming that in the 1000 years of his life the functional organization of his body was never interrupted. Following this view, the identity of his person would have remained unaltered.

If, like Glannon, we take a criterion for personal identity from the second group — in which psychological attributes are instrumental in conveying personal identity — it also appears debatable whether Methuselah 'housed' several different persons. Glannon does not explicitly say which criterion from the second group underlies his analysis. From his description of Methuselah's life, however, he appears to assume that the hundred-year old was still the same person as the child, since he can remember childhood experiences. Yet the two-hundred-year old, who cannot remember anything before his 70th birthday, is no longer personally identical to Methuselah the child. He is, however, identical in person to Methuselah the hundred-year old. Thus Glannon appears to take the following simple version of the memory criterion as a prerequisite for personal identity:

> Person P_2 is at a particular moment in time T_2 exactly the same person as person P_1 at a different particular moment in time T_1 if P_2 can remember the experiences had by P_1 (Gordijn, 1996).

Any evaluation of Methuselah's personal identity during his 1000-year lifespan based on this criterion is subject to the following two points of criticism: Firstly, it is a general fact that no human being — not even one under the age of 130 — can remember all the events which have ever occurred in his or her life. And secondly, this criterion lacks the characteristic of transitivity inherent to every relationship of identity.[15] The criterion selected by Glannon states that if a person P_3 can remember the experiences of a person P_2, and P_2 can remember the experiences of a person P_1, but P_3 cannot remember the experiences of P_1, then P_3 is identical to P_2, and P_2 is identical to P_1, but P_3 is *not* identical to P_1. A revised memory criterion could now be taken in reaction to these two points of criticism, stating:

---

[15] The transitivity rule states that if A and B are identical, and B and C are identical, then A and C are also identical.

> Person P_n at a point in time T_n is identical in person to a person P_1 at a point in time T_1, if P_n at the moment T_n can remember the experiences of P_{n-1} at the moment T_{n-1}, who in turn [...] and who can ultimately remember the experiences of P_1 at the moment T_1 (Gordijn, 1996).[16]

Thus a person P_n at a point in time T_n would be exactly the same person as a person P_1 at a point in time T_1 if P_n at time T_n were to be connected with the experiences of P_1 at time T_1 through a continuous chain of memories. This criterion takes into account the transitivity characteristic of identity relations. Taking this criterion for personal identity would mean, however, that the personal identity of Methuselah would remain unaltered throughout his life.

If, in addition to the special psychological connection between certain experiences and our memories of them, we now also take into account other psychological links, such as that between the intention behind a certain action and the action itself, the continuity of a human character or the link between traumatic experiences in childhood and corresponding fears, traits of personality and attitudes in adulthood, the following criterion could be formulated:

> A person P_n at a point in time T_n is exactly the same person as a person P_1 at a point in time T_1 if P_n has a certain psychological connection to P_{n-1}, who in turn [...] and who ultimately has a psychological connection to P_1 (Gordijn, 1996).

According to this criterion, P_n would be exactly the same person as P_1 if P_n were connected to P_1 by a continuous chain of psychological links. Taking this criterion for personal identity in the case of Methuselah, there does seem to have been such a continuous chain of psychological links. This would mean, however, that also with this criterion he would have remained one and the same person throughout his life. Consequently, longevity would not imply *per se* any alteration to personal identity. This exposition casts doubt on Glannon's thesis (1) that Methuselah's personal identity altered on several occasions.

Regarding Glannon's thesis (2) — as in the case of Methuselah, it would not be rational for the young person to want to have anything to do with the old human being in possession of an altered personal identity (Glannon, 2002b) — even this appears to be wrong. The the-

---

[16] The index n here refers to a random, but firmly selected, natural number.

sis contradicts our intuition and common sense. Why should it not be rational for a young person to be interested in the lives of his parents and grandparents and to want to associate with them? The latter may be different from the young person, but our common sense does not deem it irrational that he should wish to spend time with these older persons and to foster an interest in their continued existence (Harris, 2002). If it is conceivable, however, that an interest for other human beings clearly not personally identical can be fostered, then it seems *a fortiori* conceivable that one could be interested in future persons who will share the same body.

In summary then, Glannon's first thesis is doubtful and his second even seems to be wrong. This renders the conclusion he draws from his two theses — that any significant prolonging of life would, as in the case of Methuselah, be undesirable — likewise doubtful. The problem of undesirable alterations to personal identity as a consequence of longevity is thus revealed to be a pseudo-problem.

8.4.3 *Undesirable effects in the longer term*

Rising costs for nursing and medical care

A first conceivable longer-term effect of interventions to delay the biological aging process could be a potentially drastic rise in health costs for society (Chadwick, 1999). Could we ever justify such interventions in the light of the shortage of medical resources already upon us?

To further analyze this issue, we first need to distinguish between the interventions to delay the biological aging process themselves and the consequences of these interventions. In order to make a realistic estimate of the financial costs arising in conjunction with the *interventions themselves*, sufficient information about the exact procedures involved in such interventions must be gleaned. And yet this is not possible to date, since interventions have yet to be developed and performed in practice. It therefore makes little sense to speculate about the costs potentially involved in such interventions. A statement as to whether the costs of the interventions themselves could be justifiable in the light of the present shortage of medical resources is therefore not possible.

Would, on the other hand, the costs arising in conjunction with the potential *consequences* of interventions to delay the biological aging process be justifiable in the light of resource shortages? The potential consequences of such interventions may be outlined as follows: First of all, the normal lifespan of appropriately treated human beings would be lengthened. These human beings would then — depending on the extent of their longevity — make use of the healthcare system for longer.

Finances are already short in the healthcare sector today. One of the reasons for this is an increasing financial burden attributable to the necessity of nursing and caring for an increasing number of old people (Arking, 1998; Callahan, 1987; Daniels, 1988). Delaying the normal biological aging process would mean further exacerbation of the present financial shortage. In the light of this further threat to the financial situation, the introduction of interventions to manipulate the human lifespan would appear to be irresponsible, only serving to put even more strain on the system (Glannon, 2002b).

If we assume for a moment, however, that stretching the various phases of human life — childhood, youth or old age — would not significantly increase the quantity of diseases emerging during each phase, then it is conceivable that the longer period of healthcare necessary towards the end of life could be balanced out. After all, the phase in which human beings would be in full possession of their faculties and capable of working would also be prolonged. This would mean that they would also be obliged to pay health insurance premiums for longer. And this in turn could compensate for the increase in costs incurred during old age. It is thus conceivable that the consequences of interventions to delay normal biological aging could have a neutral effect on the financial situation (Harris, 2002). Any prediction at this stage of the exact consequences of such interventions for the present financial shortages within the healthcare sector would thus appear to be problematic.[17]

Medicalization of normal biological aging

If in the future it were really to become possible to delay normal biological aging using special medical interventions, it is conceivable that, in time, attitudes towards biological aging could alter in the following, undesirable way: The greater the number of people subject-

---

[17] Dwayne Banks and Michael Fossel demonstrate the complexity of this issue by referring to a scale of various factors upon which financial developments would depend if interventions to delay the biological aging process were to be performed (Banks & Fossel, 1997).

ing themselves to such medical treatment became, the more the pressure on others to do likewise would grow.[18] Without interventions to slow down the aging process, the latter would no longer be able to keep up with other members of their generation. Aging would ultimately still remain an inevitable component of human existence, and yet there would be a certain obligation to be successful in life and take all the steps available to delay old age for as long as possible. Normal biological aging could in time come to be viewed as a deficit requiring elimination. This could in turn lead to anxiety in some human beings about whether their lives are fundamentally intact. Through this medicalization of biological aging, and the development of ways to delay it, old age could even begin to be viewed as more problematic than prior to these developments.

In addition, human beings could become so caught up in the medical possibilities of delaying the biological aging process, and so obsessed with repeatedly prolonging their lifespans, that the old age still ultimately 'hitting' them eventually — intrinsically linked to life, as it seems to be, in the same way as death — could be experienced as a huge tragedy. Interventions to delay the normal biological aging process would put this experience off, maybe even several times: its ultimate arrival could be all the more terrible for it.

Social injustice

A further problem could emerge if interventions in the biological aging process should turn out to be contributing to social injustice. Social injustice arises as a result of social differences existing unfairly within a society. Nevertheless, social differences are not unfair *per se*. For example, it is often considered only fair that somebody who works harder and performs better should also earn more and be allowed to enjoy a higher standard of living. Unfair social differences only arise as a result of an ethically unjustifiable distribution of social goods such as status, prestige, money or employment.

Would interventions in the biological aging process bring about an unjust distribution of social goods? Two conceivable scenarios can be distinguished in this context: In the first, interventions to delay biological aging are reserved for a small group, that of the wealthy; in

---

[18] Always assuming that delaying normal biological aging would not negatively effect quality of life.

the second, these interventions would be available to everyone, without restriction. Within these two scenarios a further distinction is made between an *intragenerational* distribution of social goods, i.e. within a single generation, and *intergenerational* distribution, i.e. a distribution of social goods across various generations.

Scenario 1: Interventions to delay normal biological aging for a privileged few

In this scenario, only the wealthy within a society[19] would profit from the effects of interventions in the biological aging process, i.e. only those already benefitting from lofty social status, considerable power and high regard. Those at the pinnacle of their careers and with influential positions within society would be the very people in a position to delay their biological aging. Such interventions would thus clearly provoke a more *unequal* distribution of social goods at an *intragenerational* level. By prolonging the lifespans of those already privileged within society, these interventions would facilitate a further reinforcement and improvement of these people's already outstanding social and professional standing.

Can this intragenerationally unequal distribution of goods also be characterized as *unjust*, though? To answer this, we need to distinguish between two types of social goods which a person can acquire in the course of his or her life. The first type includes social goods which we enjoy having, but which hardly leave behind any permanent effects, for example a meal in a restaurant, a holiday, the purchase of art or a visit to a concert. These goods are chiefly sought after and enjoyed for the intrinsic value associated with them.[20] The second type includes social goods which possess not only an intrinsic, but also an extrinsic value, for example a solid education, strong health or a good upbringing.

Goods in this second category can be enjoyed for their own sake; having them also increases one's chances of acquiring other social goods. In a sense they function as catalysts to social success. Politicians often strive for a more or less equal distribution within society of the goods within this second category, in other words a distribu-

---

[19] In this context society can be taken to mean either a national or a global entity.

[20] Elsewhere (see 5.2.2) it has already been explained that there is a difference between entities worth striving for in their own right — e.g. happiness or justice — and others which primarily serve as the means to realizing other desirable ends, and which are thus in themselves indirectly desirable.

tion independent of income, social status, etc. Attempts at this kind of distribution can be perceived in healthcare and education, for example. Social policy is based on the ideal of equal opportunity with regard to social success, as well as the elementary moral idea of solidarity towards the weaker members of society.

Interventions to delay the normal biological aging process could be counted as social goods belonging to the second category. Delaying the aging process would facilitate a better education, for example. There would be more time to make career preparations. The time required to develop a career and to enjoy the success a career can bring would also be stretched. Once again, making such interventions available to just a small social elite would exacerbate the unequal distribution of many different social goods. And as this exacerbation would be diametrically opposed to the principles of solidarity and equal opportunity, it actually would be unjust. The intragenerational distribution of goods within the first scenario would thus be problematic regarding social justice (cf. Harris, 2002).

What effect would reserving interventions in the biological aging process for a wealthy elite have on the *intergenerational* distribution of social goods? One immediate consequence would be that the first generation (G_1) to subject itself to age-related interventions would be able to maintain its lofty social status for longer than the generation prior to the existence of such possibilities (G_0). As a logical result, the elite of the second generation (G_2) would be deprived of the top positions for longer. The elite of G_2 would, however — provided it also subjected itself to age-related interventions — still have the chance at a later age to assume the top functions and keep them for a while. Without such interventions this would be more or less impossible. The disadvantages of a longer waiting period would thus be relativized. This means that, intergenerationally, there would be one unique chance to gain personal advantage from this distribution of social goods, and that would be for the elite of G_1 — profiting from age-related interventions — over the elites of both G_0 and G_2. Compared with G_0, G_1 could occupy the top jobs for longer. In addition, G_1 would achieve these lofty positions far earlier on than G_2. Precisely which generation would benefit from this cited advantage would depend on which generation were alive at the moment when truly effective longevity-achieving techniques are invented. In the above example this would 'coincidentally' be G_1. Since this advantage would come from historical contingency, and not be earned in any way, it could be perceived as unjust. This would mean a problem of social justice with regard to the intergenerational distribution of social goods between G_1 and the remaining generations. Among the generations succeeding G_2 there would no longer be any significant differences and thus no social injustice. All these later generations would assume the top jobs equally late in life, all then being able to keep them for longer.

Scenario 2: Interventions to delay normal biological aging for the
           public at large

In a scenario where interventions in the biological aging process would be accessible to the entire population, there would be no exacerbation of *intragenerational* social differences regarding the distribution of social goods. Here any interested individual would have the chance to undergo such an intervention and profit from it accordingly. Thus no social injustice would be created by these interventions.

As far as the *intergenerational* distribution of social goods is concerned, the situation would be the same as in the first scenario. The first generation (G_1) to undergo age-related interventions would, as a result of being able to assume the top positions in society at a relatively young biological age and then being able to keep them for a very long time, have a one-off advantage over the following generation (G_2). G_2 could also undergo corresponding interventions and thus relativize this disadvantage, but a certain degree of social injustice would nevertheless remain. This would no longer be the case with the generation following G_2, however, as there would be no significant difference between it and G_2 regarding the distribution of social goods.

In conclusion, then, interventions in the biological aging process would only entail a clearly unjust distribution of social goods if reserved exclusively for a wealthy elite. It is probable, however, that — at least at the beginning — this new technology will only be available to certain powerful and rich elites (Chadwick, 1999; Harris, 2002; Hayflick, 2000; Sills et al. 2001). The problem of social injustice potentially emerging as this technology is applied should therefore be taken seriously.

Overpopulation

It is feared by some that a practice of intervening in the biological aging process could exacerbate the overpopulation problem (Glannon, 2002b). The so-called overpopulation problem is a complex phenomenon. Increasing world population figures are only one aspect of many.[21] Another aspect is the unequal distribution of wealth on our planet. The next important aspect is the way in which man might shape his future (further expansion *versus* stabilization of present affluence levels). Future developments in science and technology also play a crucial role. They would determine, for example, how many people with acceptable living standards the Earth could tolerate — without being badly damaged. With new technologies, mankind might one day be in a position to increase global production of foodstuffs. If progress in science and technology were to lead to significantly neater and more efficient production than we have now, we could be optimistic about the future. If, on the other hand, science and technology were not to progress sufficiently, and if mankind were to consume the resources available at the same rate as today, then we might need to fear serious shortages. The following exposition disregards all these additional aspects, however, and concentrates exclusively on the aspect of increasing world population figures.

An increase (or decrease) in world population depends, among other things, on three factors: (1) expected trends regarding an increase or decrease, (2) the effect which potential future interventions in the biological aging process could have on the human lifespan and (3) the spread of such interventions throughout the world.

The following can be said about the first factor: With regard to future trends regarding an increase or decrease in world population figures, the apocalyptic prophecies made by the *Club of Rome* in the early 1970s have been proven false. Over the past few decades the population has not increased at the same rate as expected. On the contrary: in 2000 the population was 6.1 (U.S.) billion, and there was a population growth decrease of 1.2% (United Nations, 2001). It is not unlikely that population growth could eventually come to a standstill (Lutz et al. 2001; United Nations, 1998). The UNO, for example, expects the world population to stabilize after 2200. It estimates that the population at that time will amount to somewhat over 10 (U.S.) billion (United Nations, 1998). The empirical observation that couples in technologically advanced countries tend to have fewer children plays a role in this trend. As social and technological developments increase, the number of children per family tends to decrease. This process is especially noticeable in Western industrial nations.

Some of these states already have negative population growth. According to Lutz et al. (2001) there is an 85% chance that world population growth will come to a standstill before the end of this century. The probability of there not being more than 10 (U.S.) billion people in the world when this happens is estimated by Lutz et al. at 60%. And they even believe there to be a 15% chance that the total could be below that of the current population figures (Lutz et al. 2001).

The second factor playing a role in increasing world population figures was the effect on the human lifespan of interventions to delay the biological aging process. If the human lifespan were only to lengthen slightly as a result, the effect on the overpopulation problem would be marginal. If, on the other hand, these interventions were to prolong the human lifespan radically — from 120 years maximum to 180 years or more — then the effect would be very noticeable indeed.

With regard to the last factor, a spreading of interventions to delay biological aging throughout the world, we may assume that this would be relatively sparse to start with. And if this development were to remain restricted to a small, wealthy elite able to afford the interventions (Chadwick, 1999; Harris, 2002; Hayflick, 2000; Sills et al. 2001), the overpopulation problem would hardly be exacerbated.[22]

All in all, it is difficult to evaluate the extent to which interventions in the biological aging process would really increase world population figures and thus potentially constitute an exacerbation of the world overpopulation problem. We may assume, however, that such interventions, at least at the beginning, would not lead to extreme longevity, and that in relative terms they would not be widespread. Thus the consequences of intervening in the biological aging process do not seem to represent an insurmountable difficulty in conjunction with the complex problem of world overpopulation.

Increasing numbers of harmful genes in the gene pool

Walter Glannon (2002a) believes it possible that human longevity, achieved through the genetic manipulation of many successive gen-

---

[21] Incidentally, this one aspect might not even be an insurmountable problem. Already it would be possible, at least technically, to feed and house the entire world population.

[22] Finally, if the longevity interventions were to be performed during a phase in people's lives where they were still largely healthy, they could also remain productive and serve society for longer (Harris, 2002).

erations, could lead to an increase in genes within the gene pool which could be seriously harmful to man, also early on in life.

Glannon's view is supported by ideas put forward by Nesse and Williams (1994) on the role played in the aging process by pleiotropic genes — i.e. single genes producing multiple effects. To illustrate this idea, the authors cite the example of a gene which, on the one hand, alters calcium metabolism and induces bones to heal faster, but, on the other hand, also leads to a slow and continual depositing of calcium in the human arteries. This pleiotropic gene is thus advantageous to man at the early stages of his life; as he grows older, the same gene begins to cause damage. According to Nesse and Williams, natural selection favors such 'two-sided' genes to the same extent as those without this significant disadvantage. This is due to the fact that the pressure behind natural selection is geared exclusively to the phase relevant to the transferal of genes — i.e. until the end of the human reproductive phase. During this relatively early phase, possession of the cited pleiotropic gene is advantageous. It is irrelevant to natural selection that this gene begins to trigger negative processes later on in life. These processes pose no threat to the passing on of genes to the next generation (Nesse & Williams, 1994).

Bearing this in mind, Glannon believes the following problematic development to be possible. If we assume that germ line genome modifications (see Chapter 7) were to be performed in many people for the purposes of longevity over several generations, then new genes with an advantageous effect in later life — significant longevity — would continually be entering the gene pool. Genes with such effects would thus be more or less 'artificially selected' over generations. But these selected genes could also include pleiotropic genes, which in addition to the positive effect of longevity — the reason behind the 'artificial selection' — could also have negative effects in the early stages of human life.

Since 'two-sided' genes are not detected and discarded during the process of artificial selection, more and more of them could enter the gene pool from one generation to the next. This would mean, however, that slowly but surely, from generation to generation, increasing numbers of health problems could occur in the early stages of life, maybe even including premature death. The first few generations — to implement the modifications — might gain considerable benefits from artificial selection to prolong the human lifespan; this same practice could mean increasing burdens on the generations to follow,

though, with health problems in early life and maybe even premature death to contend with. It would be unfair for early generations
to benefit themselves at such a high price to later generations (Glannon, 2002a).

This problem put forward by Glannon is speculative. It is not yet
known whether — as Glannon maintains in his hypothesis — artificially selected genes really would include pleiotropic genes with the
unpleasant side-effects cited. There are simply no data available
regarding potential damage to young people in far-off generations to
back up this hypothesis. It is also conceivable that any such defects
could be eliminated with the help of future technologies not yet
developed (Harris & Holm, 2002). Overall this does not then seem to
be an insurmountable problem.

8.5 Conclusion

Evaluation of the research field objectives

Once again, we shall first look at the results of the analysis with
regard to whether the two objectives underlying this research field —
'increasing the preventive and therapeutic options available' and
'extending the maximum lifespan' — really would be desirable. The
analysis reveals the following: The first objective is extrinsically valuable. Improved prevention and therapy of age-related diseases available as a result of interventions in the normal biological aging
process would contribute to human health and well-being, as well as
the avoidance of suffering and premature death. Thus the first of
these two objectives really is desirable, especially bearing in mind
that human beings are growing older all the time.

By contrast, the second objective — extending the maximum
lifespan — is only a desirable objective *prima facie*. On closer observation, the analysis reveals that the true motive behind this desire
for longevity is the complex problem of human attitudes to mortality. This problem cannot be solved simply by extending the maximum lifespan a little further, and then a little more. In addition, it
would not appear desirable to suppress the essential issue surrounding the meaning of life — something which could well result
from repeatedly putting off death — in the light of the fact that
death would still inevitably come eventually. And there would be
no advance guarantee that, following an intervention to prolong

life, the quality of that life would remain acceptable. These considerations mean that this second objective must be regarded as not clearly desirable.

Contribution of the research field to realizing the objectives

The results of the analysis reveal the following regarding the contribution of the research field to realizing the two objectives: First of all, all possible approaches to influencing the biological aging process known to date are all still very hypothetical. It is not at all sure whether they could ever be realized. In addition, a complete and uniform theory regarding biological aging still does not exist. And it is not at all clear whether one will ever be developed. The probability of the theoretical approaches currently available ever being put into practice is impossible to calculate.

The probability of biogerontological knowledge increasing, on the other hand, is high. It is therefore justified, or at least in theory, to assume that controlled interventions in the biological aging process could in time become practicable. This would mean that — at least in theory — it might one day be possible with the help of such interventions to increase the preventive and therapeutic options available, as well as to extend the maximum lifespan. At the current time, a real contribution of this research field to realizing these two objectives is, however, uncertain.

Ethical problems

Concerning the ethical justifiability of the various problems potentially associated with interventions in the biological aging process, the analysis reveals the following: Problems obstructing the responsible development and appropriate use of these interventions include the risks this technology could entail. There is no real scenario yet in existence pertaining to the human experiments which would be necessary to develop this technology. This means that, to date, only hypothetical statements about conceivable risks are possible. A sound reflection on the risks involved is impossible on the basis of leading edge biogerontology.

In connection with the development of interventions in the biological aging process *to increase the preventive and therapeutic options available*, the analysis revealed neither any intrinsic problems, nor any potential negative effects in the longer term.

Problems intrinsically linked with *extending the maximum lifespan* are to be viewed in connection with the goals of medicine. Leaving aside the controversial cases in which the purpose of intervening in the biological aging process would be the avoidance of premature accidental death, the purpose of such interventions would not fall under any of the four Goals of Medicine laid down by the Hastings Center in 1996 (HC, 1996). The problem cited in the literature regarding alterations to personal identity was found by the analysis to be groundless in connection with interventions to extend the maximum lifespan.

Undesirable effects potentially occurring in the longer term in connection with repeated interventions to prolong the maximum lifespan include the problem of rising costs for nursing and care. At the present time it is difficult to predict clearly even the more immediate consequences for shortages in the healthcare sector.

Another problem is the potential onset of a medicalization process with regard to normal biological aging. This process could throw the latter into an unfavorable light, possibly leading human beings to fear that their lives are fundamentally not intact. Another consequence of this process could be that human beings become so fixed upon repeatedly prolonging their lifespans that their inevitable eventual old age hits them disproportionately hard and is viewed as a tragedy.

A regular practice of interventions to prolong the maximum lifespan could also lead to social injustice. After all, it is not improbable that only the wealthy would be in a position to afford such interventions. These interventions would only lead to a clearly unjust distribution of social goods, however, if reserved exclusively for a wealthy elite within society.

In the longer term the so-called 'overpopulation problem' could additionally become exacerbated. According to the analysis, this problem seems to be surmountable, however, at least in principle. The last potential longer-term effect cited, that of an increase in harmful genes within the gene pool, was also found to be not insurmountable.

Overall, a whole series of ethical problems is conceivable in connection with the development and application of a technology to extend the maximum lifespan. Some are not easily surmountable, in particular the problems of medicalization and social injustice. And yet, for not one of the problems analyzed can clear arguments be found to render it clearly insurmountable. Whether these problems could actually be surmounted in the future, however, cannot be said. The surmountability of the ethical problems linked to *extending the maximum lifespan* is thus uncertain. No statement is possible at this stage regarding the problem of risks potentially involved in developing a technology to intervene in the biological aging process for the purpose of *increasing the preventive and therapeutic options available*.

Ethical desirability

All in all, the following picture emerges. Of the three conditions which must be fulfilled for the further development of interventions in the biological aging process to be ethically desirable, the first is fulfilled with regard to the objective 'increasing the preventive and therapeutic options available'. Regarding the objective 'extending the maximum lifespan', however, its fulfillment is problematic. Fulfillment of the second condition is found in the analysis to be problematic for both objectives, and the same is true for the third condition.

This means that — following the criteria valid in this book — the ethical desirability of further developments to technologies for intervening in the biological aging process is questionable with regard to both objectives. The results may be summarized in the following overview:

Objective		Result regarding question no.:	Condition fulfilled:		Ethical desirability
Increasing the preventive and therapeutic options available	1	Objective really desirable	yes	1	
	2	Contribution uncertain	problematic	2	Questionable
	3	Surmounting of problems uncertain	problematic	3	
Extending the maximum lifespan	1	Objective not clearly desirable	problematic	1	
	2	Contribution uncertain	problematic	2	Questionable
	3	Surmounting of problems uncertain	problematic	3	

PART III

RESULTS

9 ANALYSIS RESULTS

The aim of this book was to develop a critique of medical utopian thought from an ethical standpoint. To this end, the author examined whether the further development of tissue engineering, bioelectronics, germ line genome modifications and interventions in the biological aging process — all fields inspiring high levels of utopian euphoria — may be viewed as ethically desirable. So how does this key issue appear now? As a reminder, in this book the further development of a research field is deemed ethically desirable if the following conditions are fulfilled:

Condition 1: The objectives behind further development of the medical research field are truly ethically desirable.

Condition 2: The advocated further development of the research field really would contribute to realizing these objectives.

Condition 3: The ethical problems involved in developing the research field further are surmountable or justifiable.

The author analyzed the four research fields to examine whether they fulfill these conditions. For each of these research fields, the following three questions were posed, corresponding to the conditions:

Question 1: Are the objectives envisaged in connection with further development of the research field truly ethically desirable?

Question 2: Would further development of the research field really contribute to realizing these objectives?

Question 3: Which ethical problems are involved in developing the research field further, and are they surmountable or justifiable?

Where the analysis reveals that all three conditions are fulfilled for a particular objective behind the medical research field in question, its further development is deemed principally ethically desirable with regard to this one objective. If the results of the analysis reveal the fulfillment of one or more of the three conditions to be problematic regarding the objective in question, however, then the ethical desirability of developing this field further is evaluated as questionable with regard to this particular objective. And if just one of the three conditions is found to be not fulfilled for the objective in question, the further development of the research field is deemed ethically undesirable with regard to that particular objective.

9.1 Overview of the results

The analysis of these questions with regard to all four research fields produced a multitude of different answers. For purposes of clarity, the results are summarized below in a tabular overview. They are ordered according to research field and objective.

Objective		Result regarding question no.:	Condition fulfilled:		Ethical desirability
Tissue engineering: Increasing the therapeutic options available	1	Objective really desirable	yes	1	
	2	Contribution highly probable	yes	2	principally yes
	3	Problems can be surmounted	yes	3	
	1	Objective really desirable	yes	1	
Avances in research	2	Contribution highly probable	yes	2	principally yes
	3	Problems can be surmounted	yes	3	
Bioelelectronics: Increasing the therapeutic options available	1	Objective really desirable	yes	1	
	2	Contribution highly probable	yes	2	principally yes
	3	Problems can be surmounted	yes	3	
Improving sensory, motorial and cognitive abilities	1	Objective not clearly desirable	problematic	1	
	2	Contribution uncertain	problematic	2	Questionable
	3	Surmounting of problems uncertain	problematic	3	
Germ line genome modification:					
	1	Objective really desirable	yes	1	
Preventing diseases	2	Contribution uncertain	problematic	2	Questionable
	3	Surmounting of problems uncertain	problematic	3	
	1	Objective not clearly desirable	problematic	1	
Enhancing attributes	2	Contribution uncertain	problematic	2	Questionable
	3	Surmounting of problems uncertain	problematic	3	

Objective		Result regarding question no.:	Condition fulfilled:		Ethical desirability
Interventions in the biological aging process:					
Increasing the preventive and therapeutic options available	1	Objective really desirable	yes	1	
	2	Contribution uncertain	problematic	2	Questionable
	3	Surmounting of problems uncertain	problematic	3	
Extending the maximum lifespan	1	Objective not clearly desirable	problematic	1	
	2	Contribution uncertain	problematic	2	Questionable
	3	Surmounting of problems uncertain	problematic	3	

9.2 Interpretation of the results

In theory, there are three categories of response for the ethical desirability of progress in medical research fields: (1) further development is principally ethically desirable, (2) the ethical desirability is questionable, and (3) further development appears to be undesirable. What does the designation of one of these response categories signify with regard to the further development of a research field for the realization of a particular goal?

1) Further development is principally ethically desirable: If this first response category is assigned to a medical research field with regard to a particular objective, this means that further development of this field for the realization of that objective would be fundamentally welcome from an ethical point of view. This evaluation should not be taken as a *carte blanche* for unrestricted further development, however. Instead, the various ethical problems described in the analysis should be addressed before proceeding to develop the research field further in an ethically responsible manner.

This bid for caution can best be illustrated by a look at the research field of tissue engineering. The analysis found further development of this field to be principally ethically desirable with regard to both its objectives. Yet this does not automatically mean that all forms of replacement tissue or organ production would be ethically justifiable. For example, the analysis deemed as ethically problematic the use of

embryonic stem cells as starter cells. But it did reveal ethically justifiable alternatives as starter cells, for example the use of adult stem
cells.

2) The ethical desirability of further development is questionable:
The evaluation 'questionable' for the ethical desirability of further
developing a certain research field in order to attain a particular
objective should be viewed as a serious warning against further
research without due care and attention. It is not meant to suggest
that further development of the research field in question should stop
immediately and entirely. There is, however, a sliding scale for the
severity of the evaluation 'ethical desirability questionable'. If, for
example, with regard to a particular objective, the fulfillment of only
one of the three conditions has been found to be problematic, then
the criteria governing this book dictate that the ethical desirability of
further developing the research field in question in order to attain
this objective still has to be deemed questionable overall. Yet this
does not necessarily mean that all further research must be stopped
immediately. Far more, this evaluation should be interpreted as a call
to pay due thought to the fundamental problems involved. Further
development should only be stopped altogether if and when these
problems begin to grow. Only then would further development of
the research field gradually begin to lose its ethical justification altogether.

   If, on the other hand, fulfillment of *all three* conditions has been
deemed problematic regarding one of the objectives behind a
research field, then the cessation of all research activities aimed at
realizing this objective seems indicated. This result means not only
that the objective in question is not clearly desirable, but that it is also
uncertain whether this objective could ever be attained by developing the research field further, and whether the ethical problems
potentially linked with further developing the research field in order
to realize this objective would ever be justifiable. Continuation of
research activities under these circumstances would amount to entering a 'minefield'. The virtue of caution demands, however, that we
avoid minefields.

   A good example of this point is further research into germ line
genome modifications for the purpose of enhancing attributes.
According to the analysis, this objective is not clearly desirable. It is
also uncertain whether developing this research field further could

ever contribute to the enhancement of particular attributes. Last but not least, it is uncertain whether the ethical problems potentially linked to further development of this research field — e.g. concerning embryo protection or the risks involved — could ever be justifiable. For reasons of prudence, it would thus seem wise to stop the research activities within this field aimed at enhancing attributes, at least as long as ethical analysis of this research does not come up with different results.The same holds for research in bioelectronics aimed at improving sensory, motorial and cognitive abilities and research in biogerontology aimed at extending the maximum human life span.

3) Further development is ethically undesirable: If, with regard to one of its objectives, further development of a research field is found to be ethically undesirable, then there can be no doubt that research activity aimed at realizing this objective should be stopped immediately. In such a case the envisaged objective is undesirable and/or the objective cannot be realized by developing the research field further and/or the ethical problems potentially linked to a further development of the research field are insurmountable. However, in none of the research fields analyzed in this book was further development found to be ethically undesirable.

Let us conclude with the following remark about this critique of medical utopias. It addressed a selection of important medical research fields which are currently wont to inspire particular medical utopian euphoria. The analysis found that further development would only be principally ethically desirable with regard to all the envisaged objectives for just one of these fields, namely tissue engineering. Concerning the research field of bioelectronics, further development is only principally ethically desirable for one of its objectives, namely 'increasing the therapeutic options available'. And concerning the remaining research fields analyzed, germ line genome modifications and interventions in the biological aging process, the ethical desirability of further development was found to be questionable for all the objectives analyzed.

This means that the utopian euphoria currently greeting decisions to take medical research projects further is not a suitable yardstick. And yet it does not render the mere existence of utopian enthusiasm towards medical progress totally worthless. One euphoric advocate will not necessarily cause developments to take a sudden and dangerous turn. Utopian euphoria therefore should not be banned from the medical field altogether. On the contrary: it even fulfills an important function within medical research. Utopian excitement constitutes an elementary motivation to develop new ideas or solutions and to explore pioneering research paths. But it must not be allowed to eclipse the ethical desirability of certain medical developments, or to render every little bit of medical progress unrestrictedly and uncritically welcome. After all, scientific progress is supposed to serve mankind, and not *vice versa*.

10 PROSPECTS

10.1 Transformatio ad optimum

For thousands of years the recuperation dogma *restitutio ad integrum* — reinstatement of human wholeness or intactness — dominated the field of medicine. In Antiquity, the *restitutio ad integrum* concept was in harmony with the idea of the healthy human organism as a well-ordered microcosm. If its order, or the configuration of its individual components, became disturbed — if, for example, the 'good ratio between the juices' became imbalanced — this caused disease. The task of medics was therefore to reinstate the original order, the *eucrasy* of the human microcosm, and thus cure the disease.

In the Middle Ages, the *restitutio ad integrum* idea was very compatible with the dominant notion of the time that God created the world and all the creatures in it according to His omniscient conceptions. Since the whole of creation was regarded as perfect — being, as it was, of divine origins — mankind, as the pinnacle of creation, was also regarded as fundamentally and naturally perfect. Medieval man viewed disease as a deviation from natural perfection. The fact that diseases could befall fundamentally perfect human beings was attributed to matters such as original sin, an erring of ways or possession by evil spirits. When human beings recovered from their sufferings, this process was equated with the resurrection of mankind on the Day of Judgement. According to Medieval precepts, earthly recovery of the perfection of human nature to some extent preempted heavenly resurrection. The *restitutio ad integrum* notion therefore had not only medical, but also theological significance.

Today the idea of reinstating the wholeness or intactness of the human body still plays a significant role. The promotion and preservation of health still count as two of the major medical goals. And yet another notion has recently entered the medical limelight, too. Beyond merely reinstating the original physical and mental states of the body, man is increasingly envisaging their optimization. The *restitutio ad integrum* dogma is thus gradually being forced to share its status in present-day medicine with the *transformatio ad optimum* idea — reshaping man to attain the optimum result or even perfection.

One reason why this new notion has surfaced within the field of medicine has to do with the altering image of mankind in the Modern Age. Whereas Ancient man was viewed as a well-ordered microcosm, and Medieval man as the pinnacle of God's creation, Modern man is seen as the flawed result of chance evolutionary processes (Olshansky et al. 2001). Bearing in mind this image of mankind as an imperfect random product, the idea of optimization, of correcting the various 'flaws' produced by evolution and improving the 'human product' with its coincidental final design, seems reasonable. A second reason for the emergence of the *transformatio ad optimum* idea is the vast extent of medical progress. In particular the various spectacular technological successes of recent times have aroused the impression that it really is possible to optimize mankind using medical means.

Mankind therefore appears to be entering a new era. The new Age will not only bear witness to a further continuation of the radical changes which have long been taking place within the natural human habitat; in addition, man will begin to use new medical technologies to change himself in accordance with his own desires. At this early stage it is impossible to say just where this medical *transformatio ad optimum* 'project' will lead man to. And yet, in his efforts at autotransformation for the purpose of enhancement, he will undoubtedly enter new territory — not only in a medical sense, but also anthropologically, psychologically and politically.

Under these unexplored circumstances, unbridled utopian euphoria would not appear to be the best basis for decision-making about the biomedical course of the future. Utopian fantasies about various optimization possibilities are often swept along by uncontrolled technical optimism. They are regularly accompanied by an uncritical certainty that the various problems potentially associated with an advocated technological development will undoubtedly be able to be solved using just that same technology.

Harboring a general dystopian mistrust, on the other hand, would hardly be helpful either. Categorical damnation of all medical and technical progress on suspicion of the existence of underlying plotting — medical and technical progress being merely the product of self-enriching capitalist and industrial machinations — could amount to throwing the baby out with the bathwater. Against a background of the equally fascinating and fearsome potential of a medical field capable of putting the *transformatio ad optimum* idea into practice, a well-researched and profound debate would be much more advisable. It is the only way in which new, *argumentatively* founded ethical concepts and parameters necessary for a future biomedical course may be developed.

The conduction of such rational debates is a key task of modern medical ethics. As further motivation for a debate of this kind, this book will conclude with two topics, the closer examination of which should play a prominent role in ethical reflection on the idea of *transformatio ad optimum*, namely improvement and posthumanity.

10.2 Improvement

The idea of human optimization and self-perfection is not new. It has been around since time immemorial. The desire to realize this notion seems to be more or less innate. What is new about the present medical *transformatio ad optimum* project is thus not the interest in self-perfection *per se*, but far more the particular approach with which man is planning to achieve it. The vehicle for attaining self-perfection is no longer primarily to be mental study or physical training, but medical intervention. Bearing this intention in mind, it would be advisable to address the following two questions without delay: (1) Which alterations to mankind would constitute a real improvement? (2) To what extent is looking to medicine as the sole vehicle for human improvement desirable?

Examination of the first issue would appear necessary for the following reason: Before man can begin to use medicine as a vehicle for his own improvement with any ethical justification, he has to possess a clear idea about the intended modifications. Such clarity presupposes an exact picture of the alterations man would need to make to himself in order to arrive at an improvement over his present manifestation. At present this exact picture is wanting, however. It is thus currently impossible to establish whether a particular envisaged human modification really would represent an improvement. For example, would it be advantageous to transfer the content of the human brain to a computer and promote its continued existence as an upload *in silico* within an artificial reality created by computers? Or would it be better to continue existing within the physical reality as a cyborg equipped with the body of a robot and sensors? Would the acquisition of a vastly improved memory or a cyberthink provision be advisable, in order to communicate invisibly with persons in far-off locations? Would the possession of superintelligence be desirable? Would the ability to see infrared light be so advantageous that it would be worth undergoing genetic manipulation in order to acquire it? Unfortunately, a detailed debate about the first issue cited above — the exact image man has of 'his own improvement' — has not even really begun yet. This will have to change if plans for medical self-perfection are to have any chance of success in the future.

One of the reasons why a debate is required on the second issue cited above is the fact that focusing exclusively on medicine as a vehicle for man's improvement could potentially have an undesirable influence on his picture of optimization and self-perfection. In order to elucidate this point, the new medical *transformatio ad optimum* project will now be compared and contrasted with an earlier project also aimed at self- perfection.

In connection with self-perfection, Ancient man operated with the regulative idea of 'becoming like God' (*homoiosis theoi*). This regulative idea originated in the teachings of the Orphic religion. According to these teachings, there is a fundamental kindred of spirits between the human and the divine. The task of the soul is to maintain this kindred during its life on Earth — i.e. during its time away from God. If it is successful in this mission, the soul can reunite with deity — its origins — once the human being it has been occupying dies. Plato was later to adopt these teachings and develop them further.[1] In his view, a human being who has become similar to God is a just human being (*Politeia* 500B-500D & 612E-613B). After all, the gods themselves are just *par excellence* (*Politeia* 352A-B). The *homoiosis theoi* imposed upon man finds its expression in the development of the virtue justice. Plato's picture of human perfection thus also included a moral component. In the further course of history, the idea of *homoiosis theoi* assumed various philosophical and theological manifestations. Remarkably, the notion of human improvement associated with *homoiosis theoi* remained firmly linked to the realization of moral virtues, just as it had been in both Plato's time and at the height of Christianity.

---

[1] According to Plato, *homoiosis theoi* can only be realized through an occupation with philosophy, by recognizing the divine in the Ideas (Phaidon 79A-84C).

Contrasting the modern medical *transformatio ad optimum* project with the much earlier project of *homoiosis theoi*, the following interesting difference becomes apparent. The latter project primarily contains moral ideals regarding improvement. By contrast, the optimization of mankind envisaged with the help of medicine as a vehicle predominantly contains amoral components. The modern project is primarily aimed at an improvement of human sensory, motorial and cognitive abilities. And yet its neglecting to address the improvement of moral qualities is hardly a surprise considering the peculiarities of the present choice of improvement vehicle. The improvement of human moral qualities, requiring a certain inner development and maturity, seems to be principally impossible with medical means.

Therefore, this particular choice of medicine as an improvement vehicle could lead to a gradual disappearance of moral qualities from man's image of self-improvement. Sensory, motorial and cognitive aspects would slowly take their place. To concentrate on the vehicle of medicine for self-optimization and self-perfection could thus well mean to neglect the moral dimension of human improvement.

10.3 Posthumanity

The second issue which should play a significant role in ethical reflection about the medical *transformatio ad optimum* project is posthumanity.[2] Man's striving to change himself according to his own wishes could ultimately lead to a situation where it is no longer fitting to speak of 'man' at all. Various recent medical utopian fantasies describe how this process could unfold. With medical help, man departs from his human existence, with all its innate weaknesses and imperfections. One example of such a fantastic surmounting of human existence would be the fusion of man and machine (Kurzweil, 1999). In another example, man is reshaped with the help of germ line genome modifications, performed consistently through successive generations (Silver, 1997). A third example is the so-called 'uploading' scenario. This procedure would involve transferring the contents of the human brain to a computer (Bostrom,

---

[2] This has increasingly been a topic of discussion over the past few years (see e.g. Fukuyama, 2002; Gray, 2001; Hayles, 1999).

2003). Using appropriately specialized nanomachines, the brain would be scanned at a sufficient resolution atom by atom. Then this information would be digitized and the neuronal networks of the brain could be implemented on an electronic medium thereby bringing into existence a software resident intelligence that could continue to exist *in saecula saeculorum*.

On the one hand, these scenarios seem extremely speculative at present. On the other hand, it seems difficult to refute the idea that in time the medical *transformatio ad optimum* project might indeed come up with highly sophisticated and drastic enhancement technologies that could change man so radically that we could no longer speak of human beings in the conventional sense. Accordingly, it would be advisable to reflect prospectively on the implications of such a development. In this context, the following two questions should be addressed in particular: (1) Which alterations would change man so radically that he could only be regarded as a posthuman being, and no longer as a human being? (2) Would it be ethically desirable for the human race to enter a posthuman existence?

Concentration on the first question would be advisable in order to create a basis for a fruitful, anticipative, ethical analysis. Without a sufficiently clear picture of what would constitute the transition from humanity to posthumanity, an ethical evaluation of this transition would hardly be possible. To date it is not sufficiently evident how exactly man would have to change before we could cease to speak of a human being at all. Clear concepts to describe the transition from humanity to posthumanity are lacking. It is also unclear which aspects of humanity — e.g. biological, psychological, sociological or political — should take priority in this description.

A critical analysis of the second question — whether it would be ethically desirable to enter a posthuman existence — is particularly indicated in the light of the following: In recent times, the prospect of mankind transforming into a posthuman race has increasingly led to widespread utopian enthusiasm. Various movements propagating a complete surmounting of human nature already exist. They include, for example, the 'transhumanists'. This group anticipates a future full of posthuman beings considerably superior to the human beings of today. Its members are already actively preparing for the radical physical, mental and social changes which they believe will occur to mankind in the near future. The number of people joining such groups has grown considerably in the last few years. Local transhumanist movements have been set up in many different countries. The remarkable thing about these transhumanistic groups is their fundamentally positive evaluation of a potential future posthuman era without having a really clear idea of what a transition to posthuman existence would itself actually involve. Quite obviously, the mere idea of some kind of radical transformation from a human to a posthuman existence is enough to inspire huge enthusiasm. One gets the impression that the supporters of this idea expect the surmounting of humanity simultaneously to mean a liberation from all the problems connected with human existence.

And yet, bearing in mind the critique of medical utopias forming the core of this book, the utopian euphoria inspired by a radical transformation of mankind would appear to be a poor yardstick for decisions to be made about future medical developments. Instead, it would seem far more necessary to reflect profoundly upon whether it is really realistic to expect a 'posthumanization' of mankind to solve all the problems accompanying human existence. On the contrary, such a development would quite probably give rise to all manner of new and previously unknown problems.

The reflection called for regarding the ethical desirability of transforming mankind into a posthuman race should first be directed at a far more precise description of the various possible transformations *en route* to a posthuman existence. The next step would be a thorough ethical analysis of the scenarios potentially created by these various transformations. Only in this way could a sound basis emerge for a critical evaluation of the ethical desirability of transforming humanity into posthumanity. This is extremely important. It affects the future of the entire human race. In the light of the exponential acceleration of technological and scientific progress, choosing to ignore its significance could mean a danger of running, unprepared, full-tilt into unwanted new developments.

LITERATURE

Abkowitz JL, Can Human Hematopoietic Stem Cells become Skin, Gut, or Liver Cells? *The New England Journal of Medicine* 2002; 346(10): 770-772.

Achterhuis H, *De erfenis van de utopie*. Amsterdam: Ambo, 1998a.

Achterhuis H, The Courage to be a Cyborg. *Research in Philosophy and Technology* 1998b; 17: 9-24.

Agius E, Obligations of Justice towards Future Generations: A Revolution in Social and Legal Thought. In: Agius E & Busuttil S (eds.), *Future Generations and International Law*. London: Earthscan Publications Ltd., 1998a: 3-12.

Agius E, Patenting Life: Our Responsibilities to Present and Future Generations. In: Agius E & Busuttil S (ed.), *Germ-Line Intervention and Our Responsibilities to Future Generations*. Dordrecht/Boston/London: Kluwer Academic Publishers, 1998b: 67-84.

Agius E & Busuttil S (eds.), *Germ-Line Intervention and Our Responsibilities to Future Generations*. Dordrecht/Boston/London: Kluwer Academic Publishers, 1998a.

Agius E & Busuttil S (eds.), *Future Generations and International Law*. London: Earthscan Publications Ltd., 1998b.

Ahlert G, Biogerontologie: Stand und aktuelle Entwicklungen. *Zeitschrift für Gerontologie und Geriatrie* 1999; 32(2): 112-123.

Akins RE, Can Tissue Engineering mend Broken Hearts? *Circulation Research* 2002; 90(2): 120-122.

Allard M, Lebre V, Robine JM, Calment J, *Jeanne Calment: From Van Gogh's Time to Ours: 122 Extraordinary Years*. New York: W.H. Freeman & Co., 1998.

Allsopp RC et al., Telomere Length predicts Replicative Capacity of Human Fibroblasts. *Proceedings of the National Academy of Sciences USA* 1992; 89: 10114-10118.

Allsopp RC et al., Telomere Shortening is associated with Cell Division *in vitro* and *in vivo*. *Experimental Cell Research* 1995; 220: 194-200.

American Association for the Advancement of Science (AAAS) & Institute for Civil Society (ICS), *Stem Cell Research and Applications. Monitoring the Frontier of Biomedical Research*. November 1999 (http://www.aaas.org/spp/dspp/sfrl/projects/stem/main.htm; site visited August 1 2005).

Anderson WF, Genetics and Human Malleability. *Hastings Center Report* 1990; 20: 21-24.

Anderson WF, A New Front in the Battle against Disease. In: Stock G & Campbell J (eds.), *Engineering the Human Germline. An Exploration of the Science and Ethics of altering the Genes We pass to Our Children.* Oxford/New York: Oxford University Press, 2000: 43-48.

Andrews L & Nelkin D, *Body Bazaar. The Market for Human Tissue in the Biotechnology Age.* New York: Crown Publishers, 2001.

Annas GJ, Caplan A & Elias S, Stem Cell Politics, Ethics and Medical Progress. *Nature Medicine* 1999; 5(12): 1339-1341.

Anonym, Genchirurgie. In: Graul EH (ed.), *Gegenwartslexikon, Band 1.* Stuttgart: Ernst Klett, 1973: 183-184.

Arking R, *Biology of Aging. Observations and Principles* (2nd Edition). Sunderland (MA): Sinauer Associates, Inc., 1998.

Atala A, Future Perspectives in Reconstructive Surgery using Tissue Engineering. *Urologic Clinics of North America* 1999; 26(1): 157-65.

Austad S, *Why We age. What Science is discovering about the Body's Journey through Life.* New York: John Wiley & Sons, Inc.,1997.

Ayer AJ, *Language, Truth, and Logic.* London: Gollancz, 1936.

Babensee JE, McIntire LV & Mikos AG, Growth Factor Delivery for Tissue Engineering. *Pharmaceutical Research* 2000 May; 17(5): 497-504.

Bacchetta MD & Richter G, Response to „Germ-Line Therapy to cure Mitochondrial Disease: Protocol and Ethics of In Vitro Ovum Nuclear Transplantation" by Donald S. Rubenstein, David C. Thomasma, Eric A. Schon and Michael J. Zinaman. *Cambridge Quarterly of Health Care Ethics* 1996; 5: 450-457.

Bacon F, The Essays [1597]. In: Pitcher J (ed.), *Francis Bacon. The Essays.* London: Penguin Books, 1985: 55-233.

Bacon F, The Advancement of Learning [1605]. In: Johnston A (ed.), *The Advancement of Learning and New Atlantis.* Oxford: Clarendon Press, 1974: 215-247.

Bacon F, Novum Organum [1620]. In: Urbach P & Gibson J (transl. & eds.), *Francis Bacon. Novum Organum.* Chicago und La Salle, Illinois: Open Court Publishing Company, 1994.

Bacon F, The New Atlantis [1627]. In: Johnston A (ed.), *The Advancement of Learning and New Atlantis.* Oxford: Clarendon Press, 1974: 1-212.

Bacon R, Opus Maius [ca. 1268]. In: Bridges JH (ed.), *The "Opus Majus" of Roger Bacon.* London: Williams and Norgate, 1900.

Badura-Lotter G, Adulte Stammzellen — die bessere Alternative? In: Oduncu F, Schroth U & Vossenkuhl W (eds.), Stammzellforschung und therapeutisches Klonen, Göttingen: Vandenhoeck & Ruprecht, 2002: 78-99.

Baguisi A et al., Production of Goats by Somatic Cell Nuclear Transfer. *Nature Biotechnology* 1999; 17(5): 456-461.

Baker M, Korean Report sparks Anger and Inquiry. *Science* 1999; 283(January 1): 16-17.

Baltes PB, Alter und Altern als unvollendete Architektur der Humanontogenese. *Zeitschrift für Gerontologie und Geriatrie* 1999; 32(6): 433-448.

Banks DA & Fossel M, Telomeres, Cancer, and Aging. Altering the Human Life Span. *JAMA* 1997; 278(16): 1345-1348.

Barbour V, The Balance of Risk and Benefit in Gene-Therapy. *The Lancet* 2000; 353: 384.

Barritt JA, Brenner CA, Malter HE & Cohen J, Mitochondria in Human Offspring derived from Ooplasmic Transplantation. *Human Reproduction* 2001; 16(3): 513-516.

Bayertz K, Drei Typen genetischer Argumentation. In: Sass HM (ed.), *Genomanalyse und Gentherapie — Ethische Herausforderungen in der Humanmedizin*. Berlin, Heidelberg, New York, London, Paris, Tokio, Barcelona: Springer, 1991: 291-316.

Bayertz K, Human Dignity: Philosophical Origin and Scientific Erosion of an Idea. In: Bayertz K (ed.), *Sanctity of Life and Human Dignity*. Dordrecht/Boston/London: Kluwer Academic Publishers, 1996: 73-90.

Beier HM, Totipotenz und Pluripotenz. Von der klassischen Embryologie zu neuen Therapiestrategien. In: Oduncu F, Schroth U & Vossenkuhl W (eds.), *Stammzellforschung und therapeutisches Klonen*, Göttingen: Vandenhoeck & Ruprecht, 2002:36-54.

Bender W, Gassen HG, Platzer K & Seehaus B (eds.), *Eingriffe in die menschliche Keimbahn. Naturwissenschaftliche und medizinische Aspekte. Rechtliche und ethische Implikationen*. Münster: agenda Verlag, 2000.

Bennet R, Antenatal Genetic Testing and the Right to remain in Ignorance. *Theoretical Medicine and Bioethics* 2001; 22: 461-471.

Berardino MA di, Ban Human Cloning. *Differentiation* 2002; 69: 147-149.

Berger EM & Gert BM, Genetic Disorders and the Ethical Status of Germ-Line Gene Therapy. *Journal of Medicine and Philosophy* 1991; 16: 667-683.

Bianco P & Robey PG, Stem Cells in Tissue Engineering. *Nature* 2001; 414: 118-21.

Billings PR, Germline Culture — The Genetics of Hubris. In: Stock G & Campbell J (eds.), *Engineering the Human Germline. An Exploration of the Science and Ethics of altering the Genes We pass to Our Children*. Oxford/New York: Oxford University Press, 2000: 127-130.

Billings PR, Hubbard R & Newman SA, Human Germline Gene Modification: A Dissent. *Lancet*. 1999; 353(May 29): 1873-1875.

Birnbacher D, Genomanalyse und Gentherapie. In: Sass HM (ed.), *Medizin und Ethik*. Stuttgart: Reklam, 1994: 212-231.

Black J, Thinking Twice about "Tissue Engineering". *Engineering in Medicine and Biology* 1997; 16(4): 102-104.

Bodnar AG et al., Extension of Life-Span by Introduction of Telomerase into Normal Human Cells. *Science* 1998; 279(January 16): 349-352.

Boer GJ, Ethical Issues in Neurografting of Human Embryonic Cells. *Theoretical Medicine and Bioethics* 1999; 20: 465-475.

Bogunia-Kubick K & Sugisaka M, From Molecular Biology to Nanotechnology and Nanomedicine. *Biosystems* 2002; 65(2-3): 123-138.

Bonnicksen AL, The Politics of Germline Therapy. *Nature Genetics* 1998a; 19: 10-11.

Bonnicksen AL, Transplanting Nuclei between Human Eggs: Implications for Germ-Line Genetics. *Politics and the Life Sciences* 1998b; 17(3): 3-10.

Bostrom N, *Transhumanism FAQ.* 2003 (http://transhumanism.org/index.php/WTA/faq/; site visited August 1 2005).

Both NJ de, Therapeutisch kloneren: nog verre van toepasbaar. *Nederlands Tijdschrift voor Geneeskunde* 2001; 145(44): 2111- 2115.

Bouma H, Ethical Considerations in Human Cloning. *Surgery* 1999; 125(5): 468-470.

Bova B, *Immortality. How Science is extending your Life Span — And changing the World.* New York: Avon Books, Inc., 1998.

Braddock M, Houston P, Campbell C & Ashcroft P, Born again Bone: Tissue Engineering for Bone Repair. *News in Physiological Sciences* 2001 Oct; 16: 208-13.

Brenner CA, Barritt JA, Willadsen S & Cohen J, Mitochondrial DNA Heteroplasmy after Human Ooplasmic Transplantation. *Fertility and Sterility* 2000; 74(3): 573-578.

Brin D, *The Transparent Society. Will Technology force Us to choose between Privacy and Freedom?* Reading, Massachusetts: Perseus Books, 1998.

Brindley GS & Lewin WS, The Sensations produced by Electrical Stimulation of the Visual Cortex, *Journal of Physiology* 1968; 196: 479-493.

Brown KS, Are You Ready for a New Sensation? *Spektrum der Wissenschaft* 1999; Sonderheft 4: 38-43.

Brüske M, Der „therapeutische Imperativ" als ethische und sozialethisches Problem. Zur Gefährdung der Würde des Menschen durch die Totalisierung einer „Ethik des Heilens" am Beispiel der Debatte um „therapeutischen Klonen" und verbrauchende Embryonenforschung. *Zeitschrift für medizinische Ethik* 2001; 47: 259-275.

Buchanan A, Brock DW, Daniels N & Wikler D, *From Chance to Choice. Genetics & Justice.* Cambridge: Cambridge University Press, 2000.

Bulfinch T, *The Complete and Unabridged Bulfinch's Mythology.* New York: Modern Library, 1998

Byrne JA & Gurdon JB, Commentary on Human Cloning. *Differentiation* 2002; 69:154-157.

Callahan D, *Setting Limits: Medical Goals in an Aging Society.* New York: Simon & Schuster, 1987.

Callahan D, *What Kind of Life: The Limits of Medical Progress*. Washington D.C.: Georgetown Press, 1990.

Callahan D, *False Hopes. Why America's Quest for Perfect Health is a Recipe for Failure*. New York: Simon & Schuster, 1998.

Callahan S, The Ethical Challenge of the New Reproductive Technology. In: Monagle JF & Thomasma DC (eds.), *Medical Ethics. A Guide for Health Professionals*. Rockville Maryland, AN Aspen, 1988: 26-37.

Campanella T, La Città del Sole [1623]. In: Van Heck P (transl. & ed.), *De Zonnestad*. Baarn: Ambo, 1989.

Campbell J & Stock G, A Vision for Practical Human Germline Engineering. In: Stock G & Campbell J (eds.), *Engineering the Human Germline. An Exploration of the Science and Ethics of altering the Genes We pass to Our Children*. Oxford/New York: Oxford University Press, 2000: 9-24.

Capecchi MR, Human Germline Therapy. How and Why. In: Stock G & Campbell J (eds.), *Engineering the Human Germline. An Exploration of the Science and Ethics of altering the Genes We pass to Our Children*. Oxford/New York: Oxford University Press, 2000: 31-42.

Caplan AL, *If I were A Rich Man could I buy A Pancreas? And Other Essays on the Ethics of Health Care*. Bloomington and Indianapolis: Indiana University Press, 1992.

Carnes BA, Olshansky SJ, Gavrilov L, Gavrilova N & Grahn D, Human Longevity: Nature vs. Nurture — Fact or Fiction. *Perspectives in Biology and Medicine* 1999; 42(3): 422-441.

Carper J, *Stop aging Now! The Ultimate Plan for staying Young and Reversing the Aging Process*. New York: Harper Perennial, 1996.

Carrel A & Ebeling H, Age and Multiplication of Fibroblasts. *Journal of Experimental Medicine* 1921; 34: 599-623.

Cavazzana-Calvo M et al., Gene Therapy of Human Severe Combined Immunodeficiency (SCID)-X1 Disease. *Science* 2000; 288: 669-672.

Chadwick R, Ageing and Autonomy: The Case for Genetic Enhancement. In: Lesser AH (ed.), *Ageing, Autonomy and Resources*. Aldershot/Brookfield/Singapore/Sydney: Ashgate, 1999: 35-50.

Chapekar MS, Tissue Engineering: Challenges and Opportunities. *Journal of Biomedical Materials Research* 2000; 53(6): 617-20.

Check E, Regulators split on gene therapy as patient shows signs of cancer. *Nature* 2002; 419(6907): 545-546.

Check E, Second cancer case halts gene-therapy trials. *Nature* 2003; 421(6921): 305.

Chopra D, *Grow Younger, live Longer: 10 Steps to reverse Aging*. New York: Harmony Books, 2001.

Cibelli JB, Kiessling AA, Cunnif K, Richards C, Lanza RP & West MD, Somatic Cell Nuclear Transfer in Humans: Pronuclear and Early Embryonic Development. *The Journal of Regenerative Medicine* 2001; 2:

25-31 (http://www.bedfordresearch.org/articles/cibelli_jregenmed. pdf; site visited August 1 2005).

Cibelli JB, Lanza RP & West MD, The first Human Cloned Embryo. *Scientific American* 2002; 286(1): 43-49.

Clark WR, *A Means to an End. The Biological Basis of Aging and Death.* Oxford & New York: Oxford University Press, 1999.

Clynes ME & Kline NS, Cyborgs and Space. *Astronautics* 1960; (September): 26-27 & 74-75.

CNN, 'Cyborg' technology designed to make U.S. soldiers more effective. *CNN.COM*, 2000 (http://www.cnn.com/2000/TECH/ computing/08/10/computer.soldiers.ap/; site visited August 1 2005).

Cohen J & Tomkin G, The Science, Fiction, and Reality of Embryo Cloning. *Kennedy Institute of Ethics Journal* 1994; 4: 193-204.

Cohen J, Scott R, Schimmel T, Levron J & Willadsen S, Birth of Infant after Transfer of Anucleate Donor Oocyte Cytoplasm into Recipient Eggs. *The Lancet* 1997; 350(July 19): 186-187.

Colman A & Kind A, Therapeutic Cloning: Concepts and Practicalities. *Trends in Biotechnology* 2000; 18: 192-196.

Condorcet, Esquisse d'un tableau historique des progrès de l'esprit humain [1795]. In: Pons A (ed.), *Esquisse d'un tableau historique des progrès de l'esprit humain suivi de Fragment sur l'Atlantide.* Paris: Flammarion, 1988: 79-296.

Congregatie voor de Geloofsleer (CvdG), Donum Vitae. *Archief van de Kerken* 1987; 42: 353-379.

Connors MM, Harrison AA & Summit J, Crew Systems: Integrating Human and Technical Subsystems for the Exploration of Space. *Journal of Behavioral Science* 1994; 39: 183-213.

Coors ME, Therapeutic Cloning: From Consequences to Contradiction. *Journal of Medicine and Philosophy* 2002; 27(3): 297-317.

Council of Europe, *Convention for the Protection of Human Rights and Dignity of the Human Being with regard to the Application of Biology and Medicine: Convention on Human Rights and Biomedicine.* Oviedo, 1997.

Council of Europe. Parliamentary Assembly. *Recommendation 934 on Genetic Engineering,* 1982.

Cristofalo VJ, On Models and the Study of Senescence: Reflections on the State of Biogerontology and a Farewell. *Journal of Gerontology* 1991; 46(6): B207-B208.

Crommentuyn R, Medische technologie en taalstrijd. *Medisch Contact* 2000; 55(51/52): 1849-1851.

Crouch RA, Letting the Deaf be Deaf. Reconsidering the Use of Cochlear Implants in Prelingually Deaf Children. *Hastings Center Report* 1997; 27(4): 14-21.

Curtis A & Riehle M, Tissue Engineering: The Biophysical Background. *Physics in Medicine and Biology* 2001; 46(4): R47-65.

D'mello NP, Childress AM, Franklin DS, Kale SP, Pinswasdi C & Jazwinski SM, Cloning and Characterization of *LAG1*, a Longevity-assurance Gene in Yeast. *The Journal of Biological Chemistry* 1994; 269(22): 15451-15459.

Daele W van den, Genetische Rationalisierung und Grundrechtschutz. Verfassungspolitische Aspekte der Anwendung der Genetik auf den Menschen. In: Steger U, (ed.), *Die Herstellung der Natur. Chancen und Risiken der Gentechnologie*. Bonn: Verlag Neue Gesellschaft, 1985: 135-149.

Dahse R, Fiedler W & Ernst G, Telomers and Telomerase: Biological and Clinical Importance. *Clinical Chemistry* 1997; 43(5): 708-714.

Dancy J, *Moral Reasons*. Oxford: Blackwell Publishers Ltd., 1993.

Daniels N, *Am I My Parents' Keeper? An Essay on Justice between the Young and the Old*. New York/Oxford: Oxford University Press, 1988.

Denker H-W, Embryonic Stem Cells: An Exciting Field for Basic Research and Tissue Engineering, but also an Ethical Dilemma? *Cells Tissues Organs* 1999; 165: 246-249.

Denker H-W, Forschung an embryonalen Stammzellen. Eine Diskussion der Begriffe Totipotenz und Pluripotenz. In: Oduncu F, Schroth U & Vossenkuhl W (eds.), Stammzellforschung und therapeutisches Klonen, Göttingen: Vandenhoeck & Ruprecht, 2002:19-35.

Dertouzos ML, *What will be. How the New World of Information will change our Lives*. New York: Harper Collins, 1997.

Desai TA, Micro- and Nanoscale Structures for Tissue Engineering Constructs. *Medical Engineering and Physics* 2000 Nov; 22(9): 595-606.

Descartes R, Discours de la méthode pour bien conduire sa raison et chercher la vérité dans les sciences [1637]. In: Adam C & Tannery P (eds.), *Oevres de Descartes* (13 Bände). Paris: Léopold Cerf, 1897-1913, Band 6.

Descartes R, Principes de la philosophie [1647]. In: Adam C & Tannery P (eds.), *Oevres de Descartes* (13 Bände). Paris: Léopold Cerf, 1897-1913, Band 9 II.

Deutsche Forschungsgemeinschaft (DFG), *Empfehlungen der Deutschen Forschungsgemeinschaft zur Forschung mit menschlichen Stammzellen*, 2001 (http://www.dfg.de/; site visited August 1 2005).

Djourno A & Eyries C, Prothèse auditive par excitation électrique à distance du nerf sensorial à l'aide d'un bobinage inclus à demeure. *Presse Médicale* 1957; 65(63): 1417.

Dobelle WH, Willem J. Kolff and Artificial Vision for the Blind. *Artificial Organs* 1998; 22(11): 966-968.

Dobelle WH, Artificial Vision for the Blind by connecting a Television Camera to the Visual Cortex. *ASAIO Journal American Society for Artificial Internal Organs* 2000; 46(1): 3-9.

Dobelle WH & Mladejovsky MG, Phosphenes produced by electrical Stimulation of Human Occipital Cortex, and their Application to the Development of a Prosthesis for the Blind. *Journal of Physiology* 1974; 243: 553-576.

Dobelle WH, Mladejovsky MG & Girvin JP, Artificial Vision for the Blind: Electrical Stimulation of Visual Cortex offers Hope for a Functional Prosthesis. *Science* 1974; 183(February 1): 440-444.

Dooren P van, *Klonen. Mensen en dieren op bestelling.* Leuven: Davidsfonds, 1998.

Duffy PH, Seng JE, Lewis SM, Mayhugh MA, Aidoo A, Hattan DG, Casciano DA & Feuers RJ, The Effects of Different Levels of Dietary Restriction on Aging and Survival in the Sprague-Dawley Rat: Implications for Chronic Studies. *Aging: Clinical and Experimental Research* 2001; 13: 263-272.

Eijk WJ, Criteria voor de status van het menselijk embryo. In Eijk WJ, Lelkens JPM & Garrett P (eds.), *Het embryo iets of iemand?* Oegstgeest: Colomba, 1997: 25-37.

Engelhardt, HT, Gentherapie an menschlichen Keimbahnzellen: Kann und soll die "Schöne neue Welt" verhindert werden? In: Braun V, Mieth D & Steigleder K (eds.), *Gentechnologie. Chancen und Risiken. Ethische und rechtliche Fragen der Gentechnologie und der Reproduktionsmedizin.* München: J Schweizer Verlag, 1987: 255-262.

Ennenga G, Would Humanity be Better Off ... Or, What would it be Better For? In: Stock G & Campbell J (eds.), *Engineering the Human Germline. An Exploration of the Science and Ethics of altering the Genes We pass to Our Children.* Oxford/New York: Oxford University Press, 2000: 133-135.

Enquetekommission des deutschen Bundestages, A Report from Germany. *Bioethics* 1988; 2(3): 254-263.

Erikson S, Informed Consent and Biobanks. In: Hansson MG (ed.), *The Use of Human Biobanks. Ethical, Social, Economical and Legal Aspects.* Uppsala: Universitetstryckeriet, 2001: 41-51.

Fahy GM, Short-Term and Long-Term Possibilities for Interventive Gerontology. *Mount Sinai Journal of Medicine* 1991; 58(4): 328-340.

Faragher RCA & Kipling D, How might Replicative Senescence contribute to Human Ageing? *BioEssays* 1998; 20(12): 985-991.

Feinberg J, *Freedom and Fulfillment: Philosophical Essays.* Princeton: Princeton University Press, 1994.

Fell HB, Tissue Culture and its Contribution to Biology and Medicine. *Journal of Experimental Biology* 1972; 57: 1-13.

Ferguson J, *Utopias of the Classical World.* London: Thames and Hudson, 1975.

Fiddler M & Pergament E, Germline Gene Therapy: Its Time is Near. *Molecular Human Reproduction* 1996; 2(2): 75-76.

Fiddler M, Pergament D & Pergament E, The Role of the Preimplantation Geneticist in Human Cloning. *Prenatal Diagnosis* 1999; 19: 1200-1204.

Fink J, *Cyberseduction: Reality in the Age of Psychotechnology*. Amherst, NY: Prometheus Books, 1999.

Fletcher JC, Ethische Diskussion der Gentherapie am Menschen. In: Sass HM (ed.), *Genomanalyse und Gentherapie, Ethische Herausforderungen in der Humanmedizin*. Berlin, Heidelberg, New York, London, Paris, Tokio, Barcelona: Springer, 1991: 240-291.

Fossel M, *Reversing Human Aging*. New York: William Morrow and Company, 1996.

Fowler G, Juengst ET & Zimmerman, BK, Germ-Line Gene Therapy and the Clinical Ethos of Medical Genetics. *Theoretical Medicine* 1989; 10(2): 151-165.

Frankel MS & Chapman AR, *Human Inheritable Genetic Modifications. Assessing Scientific, Ethical, Religious, and Policy Issues*. American Association for the Advancement of Science (http://www.aaas.org/; site visited August 1 2005).

Freundel RB, Gene Modification Technology. In: Stock G & Campbell J (eds.), *Engineering the Human Germline. An Exploration of the Science and Ethics of altering the Genes We pass to Our Children*. Oxford/New York: Oxford University Press, 2000: 119-121.

Friedman CD, Future Directions in Biomaterial Implants and Tissue Engineering. *Archives of Facial Plastic Surgery* 2001; 3(2): 136-137.

Fuchs JR, Nasseri BA & Vacanti JP, Tissue Engineering: A 21st Century Solution to Surgical Reconstruction. *Annals of Thoracic Surgery* 2001; 72(2): 577-591.

Fukuyama F, *Our Posthuman Future. Consequences of the Biotechnology Revolution*. New York: Farrar, Straus & Giroux, 2002.

Fuson RH, *Juan Ponce De Leon and the Spanish Discovery of Puerto Rico and Florida*. Blacksburg, Virginia: McDonald & Woodward Publishing Company, 2000.

Gardner JW & Barlett PN, A Brief History of Electronic Noses. *Sensors and Actuators B: Chemical* 1994; 18: 211-220.

Gardner W, Can Human Genetic Enhancement be prohibited? *Journal of Medicine and Philosophy* 1995; 20: 65-84.

Gauntlett R, Cochlear Implantation is Controversial among Deaf People. *British Medical Journal* 1996; 312: 850.

Gelman R, Watson A, Bronson R & Yunis E, Murine Chromosomal Regions Correlated with Longevity. *Genetics* 1988; 118: 693-704.

Gene Therapy Clinical Trials (GTCT), Website der *Journal of Gene Medicine* (http://www.wiley. co.uk/genetherapy/clinical/; site visited August 1 2005).

Gezondheidsraad, *Cochleaire implantatie bij kinderen*. Den Haag: Gezondheidsraad, 2001a.

Gezondheidsraad, *Celkerntransplantaties bij mutaties in het mitochondriale DNA*. Den Haag: Gezondheidsraad, 2001b.

Glannon W, Extending the Human Life Span. *Journal of Medicine and Philosophy* 2002a; 27(3): 339-354.

Glannon W, Identity, Prudential Concern, and Extended Lives. *Bioethics* 2002b; 16(3): 266-283.

Glover J, *What Sort of People should there be? Genetic Engineering, Brain Control and Their Impact on our Future World*. Harmondsworth, Middlesex, England: Penguin Books, 1984.

Göpel W et al., Bioelectronic Noses: A Status Report. Part I. *Biosensors & Bioelectronics* 1998; 13(3-4): 479-493.

Gordijn B, *Die Person und die Unbestimmbarkeit ihrer Grenzen. Eine grundlegende Kritik an der Debatte über Personenidentität*. Frankfurt a. M., Bern, New York, Paris, Wien: Peter Lang, 1996.

Gordijn B, The Troublesome Concept of the Person. *Theoretical Medicine and Bioethics* 1999; 20(4): 347-359.

Gordon JW, Germline Alteration by Gene Therapy: Assessing and reducing the Risks. *Molecular Medicine Today* 1998; 4(11): 468-470.

Graumann S, *Die somatische Gentherapie. Entwicklung und Anwendung aus ethischer Sicht*. Tübingen und Basel: Francke Verlag, 2000.

Gray CH, *The Cyborg Soldier: The US Military and the Post-Modern Warrior*. In: Levidow L & Robins K (eds.), *Cyborg Worlds. The Military Information Society*. London: Free Association Press, 1989: 43-72.

Gray CH, The Culture of War Cyborgs: Technoscience, Gender, and Postmodern War. *Research in Philosophy and Technology* 1993; 13: 141-163.

Gray CH, An Interview with Manfred Clynes. In: Gray CH, Figueroa-Sarriera HJ & Mentor S (eds.), *The Cyborg Handbook*. New York & London: Routledge, 1995: 43-54.

Gray CH, *Cyborg Citizen: Politics in the Posthuman Age*. New York: Routledge, 2001.

Gray CH, Figueroa-Sarriera HJ & Mentor S (eds.), *The Cyborg Handbook*. New York & London: Routledge, 1995.

Greider CW & Blackburn EH, Telomeres, Telomerase and Cancer. *Scientific American* 1996; 280(2): 80-85.

Grey ADNJ de, Noncorrelation Between Maximum Life Span and Antioxidant Enzyme Levels Among Momeotherms: Implications for retarding Human Aging. *Journal of Anti-Aging Medicine* 2000; 3(1): 25-36.

Griffith LG & Naughton G, Tissue Engineering — Current Challenges and Expanding Opportunities. *Science* 2002; 295: 1009-14.

Grikscheit TC & Vacanti JP, The History and Current Status of Tissue Engineering: The Future of Pediatric Surgery. *Journal of Pediatric Surgery* 2002; 37(3): 277-288.

Gruman GJ, A History of Ideas about the Prolongation of Life. *Transactions of the American Philosophical Society* 1966; 56(9):1-102.

Guarente L, Link Between Aging and the Nucleolus. *Genes & Development* 1997; 11: 2449-2455.

Gustafson C-J & Kratz G, Tissue Engineering in Urology. *Current Opinion in Urology* 2001; 11(3): 275-279.

Haan G de, Gelman R, Watson A, Yunis E & Zant G van, A Putative Gene causes Variability in Lifespan Among Genotypically Identical Mice. *Nature Genetics* 1998; 19(June 19): 114-116.

Hadfield P & Marks P, Nurses get Bionic "Power Suit". *New Scientist Free Newsletter* 2001; 27 July (http://www.newscientist.com/news/print.jsp?id=ns99991072; site visited August 1 2005).

Hailer M & Ritschl D, The General Notion of Human Dignity and the Specific Arguments in Medical Ethics. In: Bayertz K (ed.), *Sanctity of Life and Human Dignity*. Dordrecht/Boston/London: Kluwer Academic Publishers, 1996, 91-106.

Hansson MG (ed.), *The Use of Human Biobanks. Ethical, Social, Economical and Legal Aspects*. Uppsala: Universitetstryckeriet, 2001.

Haraway D, Manifesto for Cyborgs: Science, Technology, and Socialist Feminism in the 1980s. *Socialist Review* 1985; 80: 65-105.

Haraway D, *Simians, Cyborgs, and Women: the Reinvention of Nature*. New York: Routledge, 1991.

Hare RM, *The Language of Morals*. Oxford: Oxford University Press, 1952.

Harley CB, Futcher AB & Greider CW, Telomeres shorten during ageing of Human Fibroblasts, *Nature* 1990; 345(May 31): 458-460.

Harris J, *The Value of Life. An Introduction to Medical Ethics*. Londen: Routledge, 1985.

Harris J, A Response to Walter Glannon. *Bioethics* 2002; 16(3): 284-291.

Harris J & Holm S, Extending Human Lifespan and the Precautionary Paradox. *Journal of Medicine and Philosophy* 2002; 27(3): 355-368.

Harrison DE & Archer JR, Natural Selection for Extended Longevity from Food Restriction. *Growth, Development & Aging* 1989; 53: 3.

Hartogh GA den, *Kun je een zygote liefhebben? Over de waarde van het leven en de grenzen van de morele gemeenschap*. Rede uitgesproken op 24 september 1993 bij de aanvaarding van het ambt van bijzonder hoogleraar in de ethische aspecten van de gezondheidszorg. Universiteit van Amsterdam. Utrecht: Stichting Socrates, 1993.

Hastings Center (HC), The Goals of Medicine. Setting New Priorities. Special Supplement. *Hastings Center Report* 1996; 26 (6): 1-27.

Haugland M & Sinkjær T, Interfacing the Body's own sensing Receptors into Neural Prosthesis Devices. *Technology and Health Care* 1999; 7(6): 393-399.

Have H ten, Medical Technology Assessment and Ethics. Ambivalent Relations. *Hastings Center Report* 1995; 25(5): 13-19.

Have H ten, Genetics and Culture: The Geneticization Thesis. *Medicine, Health Care and Philosophy. A European Journal* 2001; 4(3): 295-304.

Have H ten, Meulen R ter & Leeuwen E van, *Medische Ethiek*. Houten/Diegem: Bohn Stafleu Van Loghum, 1998.

Hayflick L, The limited *In Vitro* Lifetime of Human Diploid Cell Strains. *Experimental Cell Research* 1965; 37: 614-636.

Hayflick L, *How and Why We age*. New York: Ballantine Books, 1994.

Hayflick L, The Future of Ageing. *Nature* 2000; 408: 267-269.

Hayflick L & Moorhead PS, The Serial Cultivation of Human Diploid Cell Strains. *Experimental Cell Research* 1961; 25: 585-621.

Hayles NK, *How We Became Posthuman: Virtual Bodies in Cybernetics, Literature, and Informatics*. Chicago & London: University of Chicago Press: 1999.

Häyry M & Takala T, Genetic Information, Rights, and Autonomy. *Theoretical Medicine and Bioethics* 2001; 22: 403-414.

Healy DL, Weston G, Pera MF, Rombauts L & Trounson AO, Human Cloning 2001. *Human Fertility* 2002; 5(2): 75-77.

Heath CA, Cells for Tissue Engineering. *Trends in Biotechnology* 2000; 18: 17-19.

Heller JC, Why Dignity should not keep Us from Genetically Engineering Our Children. In: Stock G & Campbell J (eds.), *Engineering the Human Germline. An Exploration of the Science and Ethics of altering the Genes We pass to Our Children*. Oxford/New York: Oxford University Press, 2000: 135-137.

Hershenov DB, An Argument for Limited Human Cloning. *Public Affairs Quarterly* 2000; 14(3): 245-258.

Hill JR, Abnormal *in utero* Development of Cloned Animals: Implications for Human Cloning. *Differentiation* 2002; 69: 174-178.

Hillmann G & Geurtsen W, Tissue Engineering — An Exciting Future. *Clinical Oral Investigations* 2001; 5(1): 1.

Höfling, W, Verfassungsrechtliche Aspekte des so genannten therapeutischen Klonens. *Zeitschrift für medizinische Ethik* 2001; 47: 277-284.

Hofman MA, On the Presumed Coevolution of Brain Size and Longevity in Hominids. *Journal of Human Evolution* 1984; 13: 371-376.

Hogle LF, Tales From the Cryptic: Technology Meets Organism in the Living Cadaver. In: Gray CH, Figueroa-Sarriera HJ & Mentor S (eds.), *The Cyborg Handbook*. New York & London: Routledge, 1995: 203-217.

Höhn H, Genetische Manipulation am Menschen — Wiederholt sich die Geschichte? In: Bender W, Gassen HG, Platzer K & Seehaus B (eds.), *Eingriffe in die menschliche Keimbahn. Naturwissenschaftliche und medi-*

zinische Aspekte. Rechtliche und ethische Implikationen. Münster: agenda Verlag, 2000, 30-53.

Holliday R, Ageing Research in the Next Century. *Biogerontology* 2000; 1: 97-101.

Holtug N, Altering Humans — The Case for and against Human Gene Therapy. *Cambridge Quarterly of Healthcare Ethics* 1997; 6: 157-174.

Holtug N & Sandøe P, Who Benefits? Why Personal Identity does not matter in a Moral Evaluation of Germ-line Gene Therapy. *Journal of Applied Philosophy* 1996; 13(2): 157-166.

Hood L, The Human Genome Project — Launch Pas for Human Genetic Engineering. In: Stock G & Campbell J (eds.), *Engineering the Human Germline. An Exploration of the Science and Ethics of altering the Genes We pass to Our Children.* Oxford/New York: Oxford University Press, 2000: 17-24.

House WF, *Cochlear Implants: My Perspective.* AllHear, Inc. 1995 (www.serve. com/AllHear/ monographs/m-95-htm.html; site visited August 1 2005).

House WF, Opposition to the Cochlear Implant in Deaf Children. *The American Journal of Otology* 1986; 7(2): 89-92.

House WF & Urban J, Long-Term Results of Electrode Implantation and Electronic Stimulation of the Cochlea in Man. *Annals of Otology, Rhinology & Laryngology* 1973; 82: 504-517.

Howel JD, The History of Eugenics and the Future of Gene Therapy. *The Journal of Clinical Ethics* 1991; 2(4): 274-278.

Hubbard R, Germline Manipulation. In: Stock G & Campbell J (ed.), *Engineering the Human Germline. An Exploration of the Science and Ethics of altering the Genes We pass to Our Children.* Oxford/New York: Oxford University Press, 2000: 109-111.

Hughes J, Liberty, Equality, and Solidarity in Our Genetically Engineered Future. In: Stock G & Campbell J (eds.), *Engineering the Human Germline. An Exploration of the Science and Ethics of altering the Genes We pass to Our Children.* Oxford/New York: Oxford University Press, 2000: 130-133.

Huizinga J, *Herfsttij der middeleeuwen. Studie over levens- en gedachtevormen der veertiende en vijftiende eeuw in Frankrijk en de Nederlanden.* Groningen: Wolters-Noordhoff, 1985 (19te Auflage).

Human Genetics Commission (HGC), *Whose Hands on Your Genes? A Discussion Document on the Storage Protection and Use of Personal Genetic Information.* London: Human Genetics Commission, 2000 (http://www. hgc.gov.uk/; site visited August 1 2005).

Human Genetics Commission (HGC), *Inside Information. Balancing Interests in the Use of Personal Genetic Information.* London: Human Genetics Commission, 2002 (http://www.hgc.gov.uk/; site visited August 1 2005).

Hutmacher DW, Goh JC & Teoh SH, An Introduction to Biodegradable Materials for Tissue Engineering Applications. *Annals of the Academy of Medicine Singapore* 2001 Mar; 30(2): 183-191.

Hutmacher DW, Teoh SH, Zein I, Ranawake M & Lau S, Tissue Engineering Research: The Engineer's Role. *Medical Device Technology* 2000; 11(1): 33-39.

Hwang WS, Ryu YJ, Park JH, Park, ES, Lee EG, Koo JM, Jeon HY, Lee BC, Kang SK, Kim SJ, Ahn C, Hwang JH, Park KY, Cibelli, JB Moon, SY, Evidence of a Pluripotent Human Embryonic Stem Cell Line Derived from a Cloned Blastocyst. *Science* 2004; 303: 1669-1674.

Jaenisch R & Wilmut I, Developmental Biology. Don't clone Humans. *Science* 2001; 291(March 30): 2552.

Jazwinski SM, Longevity, Genes, and Aging. *Science* 1996; 273(July 5): 54-59.

Jazwinski SM, Genetics of Longevity. *Experimental Gerontology* 1998; 33(7/8): 773-783.

Jazwinski SM, Longevity, Genes, and Aging: A View provided by a Genetic Model System. *Experimental Gerontology* 1999; 34(1): 1-6.

Jeuken M, *Materie, Leven, Geest. Een wijsgerige biologie.* Assen: Van Gorcum, 1979.

Jian-Gang Z, Yong-Xing M, Chuan-Fu W, Pei-Fang L, Song-Bai Z, Nui-Fan G, Guo-Yin F & Lin H, Apolipoprotein E and Longevity among Han Chinese Population. *Mechanisms of Ageing and Development* 1998; 104: 159-167.

Jiang Y et al., Puripotency of Mesenchymal Stem Cells derived from Adult Marrow. *Nature* 2002; 418(July 04): 41-49.

Jochemsen H, Het menselijk embryo als middel. Is het tot stand brengen van menselijke embryo's ten behoeve van onderzoek geoorloofd? *Medisch Contact* 1989; 44: 466-9.

Johnson PC, The Role of Tissue Engineering. *Advances in Skin & Wound Care* 2000; 13(2 Suppl.): 12-14.

Johnson TE, Lithgow GJ & Murakami S, Hypothesis: Interventions that increase the Response to Stress offer the Potential for Effective Life Prolongation and Increased Health. *Journal of Gerontology: Biological Sciences* 1996; 51A(6): B392-B395.

Johnson TE, Cypser J, De Castro E, De Castro S, Henderson S, Murakami S, Rikke B, Tedesco P & Link C, Gerontogenes mediate Health and Longevity in Nematodes through increasing Resistance to Environmental Toxins and Stressors. *Experimental Gerontology* 2000; 35: 687-694.

Johnson TE, Deqing W, Redeco P, Dames S & Vaupel JW, Age-Specific Demographic Profiles of Longevity Mutants in *Caenorhabditis elegans* show Segmental Effects. *Journal of Gerontology: Biological Sciences* 2001; 56A(8): B331-B339.

Jonas H, *Technik, Medizin und Ethik. Zur Praxis des Prinzips Verantwortung*. Frankfurt am Main: Suhrkamp, 1985.

Juengst ET, Germ-Line Gene Therapy: Back to Basics. *Journal of Medicine and Philosophy* 1991; 16: 586-592.

Juengst ET, Can Enhancement be distinguished from Prevention in Genetic Medicine? *Journal of Medicine and Philosophy* 1997; 22: 125-142.

Juengst ET, What does enhancement mean? In: Parens E (ed.), *Enhancing Human Traits. Ethical and Societal Implications*. Washington, D.C.: Georgetown University Press, 1998: 29-47.

Juengst ET & Fossel M, The Ethics of Embryonic Stem Cells — Now and Forever, Cells Without End. *JAMA* 2000; 284(24): 3180-3184.

Kaku M, *Visions. How Science will revolutionize the 21ˢᵗ Century*. New York: Anchor Books/Doubleday, 1997.

Kant I, Kritik der praktischen Vernunft [1788]. In: Vorländer K (ed.), *Immanuel Kant. Kritik der praktischen Vernunft*. Hamburg: Felix Meiner Verlag, 1985.

Kass LR, *Toward a More Natural Science. Biology and Human Affairs*. New York: The Free Press, 1985.

Kass LR, Why we should ban Human Cloning Now. Preventing a Brave New World. *The New Republic* 2001; 224(May 21): 30-39.

Kato Y et al., Eight Calves cloned from Somatic Cells of a Single Adult. *Science* 1998; 282(December 11): 2095-2098.

Kay MA, et al., Evidence for Gene Transfer and Expression of Blood Coagulation Factor IX in Patients with Severe Haemophilia B treated with an AAV Vector. *Nature Genetics* 2000; 24: 257-261.

Kielstein R & Sass H-M, From Wooden Limbs to Biomaterial Organs: The Ethics of Organ Replacement and Artificial Organs. *Artificial Organs* 1995; 19(5), 475-480.

Kim HW & Han CD, An Overview of Cartilage Tissue Engineering. *Yonsei Medical Journal* 2000; 41(6): 766-773.

Kim J-H et al., Dopamine Neurons derived from Embryonic Stem Cells function in an Animal Model of Parkinson's Disease. *Nature* 2002; 418(July 04): 50-56.

Kim SS & Vacanti JP, The Current Status of Tissue Engineering as Potential Therapy. *Seminars in Pediatric Surgery* 1999; 8(3): 119-123.

Kimbrell A, *The Human Body Shop*. San Francisco: HarperCollins Publishers, 1993

Kimura KD, Tissenbaum HA, Liu Y & Ruvkun G, *daf-2*, an Insulin Receptor-Like Gene that regulates Longevity and Diapause in *Caenorhabditis elegans*. *Science* 1997; 277(August 15): 942-946.

Kind A & Colman A, Therapeutic Cloning: Needs and Prospects. *Seminars in Cell and Developmental Biology* 1999; 10: 279-286.

King TW & Patrick CW, Ethical Considerations of Tissue Engineering on Society. In: Patrick CW, Mikos AG & McIntire LV (eds.), *Frontiers in Tissue Engineering*, Houston: Pergamon, 1998: 311-340.

Kirk KL, Dietary Restriction and Aging: Comparative Tests of Evolutionary Hypotheses. *Journal of Gerontology: Biological Sciences* 2001; 56A: B123-B129.

Kirkwood TBL, How can We live Forever? *British Medical Journal* 1996; 313(7072): 1571.

Kirkwood TBL, Biological Theories of Aging: An Overview. *Aging: Clinical and Experimental Research* 1998; 10(2): 144-146.

Kirkwood TBL, *Time of Our Lives. The Science of Human Aging*. Oxford: Oxford University Press, 1999.

Kirkwood TBL & Austad SN, Why do We age? *Nature* 2000; 408(November 9): 233-238.

Klatz R & Kahn C, *Grow Young with HGH*. New York: Harper Perennial, 1998.

Klugman CM, From Cyborg Fiction to Medical Reality. *Literature and Medicine* 2001; 20(1): 39-54.

Knook DL, Oud worden als biologisch verschijnsel. In: Schouten J, Leering C & Bender J, (eds.), *Leerboek geriatrie*. Utrecht: Bohn, Scheltema & Holkema, 1989, 2-21.

Kollek R, Klonen ist Klonen — oder nicht? In: Ach JS, Brudermüller G & Runtenberg C (eds.), *Hello Dolly? Über das Klonen*. Frankfurt a. M.: Suhrkamp, 1998: 19-45.

Kooy D van der & Weiss S, Why Stem Cells? *Science* 2000; 287: 1439-1441.

Koshland DJr, Ethics and Safety. In: Stock G & Campbell J (eds.), *Engineering the Human Germline. An Exploration of the Science and Ethics of altering the Genes We pass to Our Children*. Oxford/New York: Oxford University Press, 2000: 25-30.

Kreeft P, Human Personhood begins at Conception. *Journal of Biblical Ethics in Medicine* 1990; 4: 8-11.

Krimsky S, Human Gene Therapy: Must we know where to stop before we start? *Human Gene Therapy* 1990; 1: 171-173.

Krimsky S, The Psychosocial Limits on Human Germline Modification. In: Stock G & Campbell J (eds.), *Engineering the Human Germline. An Exploration of the Science and Ethics of altering the Genes We pass to Our Children*. Oxford/New York: Oxford University Press, 2000: 104-107.

Kuitert HM, De morele status van het embryo. De pauselijke instructie *Donum Vitae*. In: Wert GMWR de & Beaufort I de (eds.), *Op de drempel van het leven. Ethische problemen rond bevruchting, abortus en geboorte*. Baarn: Ambo, 1991: 48-72.

Kumar K, *Utopia and Anti-Utopia in Modern Times*. Oxford: Basil Blackwell Ltd., 1987.

Kurzweil R, *The Age of Spiritual Machines. When Computers Exceed Human Intelligence*. New York: The Viking Press, 1999.

Kutschera F von, *Grundlagen der Ethik*. Berlin & New York: Walter de Gruyter, 1982.

Lakowski B & Hekimi S, Determination of Life-Span in *Caenorhabditis elegans* by Four Clock Genes. *Science* 1996; 272(May 17): 1010-1013.

Lane MA, Ingram DK & Roth GS, The Serious Search for an Anti-Aging Pill. *Scientific American* 2002; 278(2): 24-29.

Lange T de, Telomeres and Senescence: Ending the Debate. *Science* 1998; 279(January 16): 334-335.

Langer R & Vacanti JP, Tissue Engineering. *Science* 1993; 260: 920-926.

Langer R & Vacanti JP, Tissue Engineering: The Challenges Ahead. *Scientific American* 1999; 280(4): 86-89.

Lanza PR et al., The Ethical Validity of Using Nuclear Transfer in Human Transplantation. *JAMA* 2000; 284(24): 3175-3179.

Lanza RP, Cibelli JB & West MD, Human Therapeutic Cloning. *Nature Medicine* 1999a; 5(9): 975-977

Lanza PR, Cibelli JB & West MD, Prospects for the Use of Nuclear Transfer in Human Transplantation. *Nature Biotechnology* 1999b; 17: 1171-1174.

Lapouge G, *Utopie et Civilisations*. Paris: Flammarion, 1978.

Lappé M, Ethical Issues in Manipulating the Human Germ Line. *Journal of Medicine and Philosophy* 1991; 16: 621-639.

Larkin M, Artificial Vision Research comes into Focus. *Lancet* 2000; 355(March 25): 1080.

Layer PG, Robitzki A, Rothermel A & Willbold E, Of Layers and Spheres: The Reaggregate Approach in Tissue Engineering. *Trends in Neurosciences* 2002; 25(3): 131-134.

Lee SS & Ruvkun G, Longevity: Don't hold your Breath. Nature 2002; 418(July 18): 287-288.

Lenk C, Therapie und Enhancement. Ziele und Grenzen der modernen Medizin. Münster/Hamburg/London: Lit Verlag, 2002.

Levy N, Reconsidering Cochlear Implants: The Lessons of Martha's Vineyard. *Bioethics* 2002; 16(2): 134-152.

Lewis D, Survival and Identity. In: Rorty A (eds.), *The Identities of Persons*. Berkeley, Los Angeles und London: University of California Press, 1976: 17-40.

Lieber CM, The Incredible Shrinking Circuit. *Scientific American* 2001; 285(3): 51-56.

Lightowlers RN, Chinnery PF, Turnbull, DM & Howel N, Mammalian Mitochondrial Genetics: Heredity, Heteroplasmy and Disease. *Trends in Genetics* 1997; 13(11): 450-455.

Lin K, Dorman JB, Rodan A & Kenyon C, *daf-16:* An HNF-3/Forkhead Family Member that can function to Double The Life-Span of *Caenorhabditis elegans. Science* 1997; 278(November 14): 1319-1322.

Lin Y-J, Seroude L & Benzer S, Extended Life-Span and Stress Resistance in the *Drosophila* Mutant *Methuselah. Science* 1998; 282(October 30): 943-946.

Lippman A, Prenatal Genetic Testing and Screening: Constructing Needs and reinforcing Inequities. *American Journal of Law and Medicine* 1991; 17: 15-50.

Lizza JP, Persons and Death: What's Metaphysically Wrong with our Current Statutory Definition of Death? *Journal of Medicine and Philosophy* 1993; 18: 351-374.

Locke J, *An Essay Concerning Human Understanding* [1690]. In: Anonym (ed.), *The Works of John Locke. A New Edition, corrected. 10 volumes. London 1823.* Aalen: Scientia Verlag (Neuauflage), 1963, Band 2.

Lunshof JE, Keimbahnmodifikation — Was spricht dagegen? In: Fischer EP & Geißler E (eds.), *Wie viel Genetik braucht der Mensch? Die alten Träume der Genetiker und ihre heutigen Methoden.* Konstanz: Universitätsverlag Konstanz, 1994: 281-288.

Lutz W, Sanderson W & Scherbov S, The End of World Population Growth. *Nature* 2001; 412(August 2): 543-545.

Luyten FP, Dell'Accio F & Bari C de, Skeletal Tissue Engineering: Opportunities and Challenges. *Best practice & Research. Clinical Rheumatology* 2001; 15(5): 759-769.

Lysaght MJ & Aebischer P, Encapsulated Cells as Therapy. *Scientific American* 1999; 280(4): 52-58.

Lysaght MJ & Reyes J, The Growth of Tissue Engineering. *Tissue Engineering* 2001; 7(5): 485-493.

Maguire GQJr & McGee EM, Implantable Brain Chips? Time for Debate. *Hastings Center Report* 1999; 7: 7-13.

Mallia P & Have H ten, From What should we protect Future Generations: Germ-line Therapy or Genetic Screening? *Medicine, Health Care and Philosophy. A European Journal* 2003; 6(1) (im Druck).

Maniglia AJ et al., The Middle Ear Bioelectronic Microphone for a Totally Implantable Cochlear Hearing Device for Profound and Total Hearing Loss. *The American Journal of Otology* 1999; 20(5): 602-611.

Maniglia AJ, Murray G, Arnold JE & Ko WH, Bioelectronic Microphone Options for a Totally Implantable Hearing Device for Partial and Total Hearing Loss. *Otolaryngologic Clinics of North America* 2001; 34(2): 469-483.

Mann BK & West JL, Tissue Engineering in the Cardiovascular System: Progress Toward a Tissue Engineered Heart. *The Anatomical Record* 2001; 263(4): 367-371.

Mann S, Wearable Computing: A First Step toward Personal Imaging. *IEEE Computer* 1997; 30(3), 25-31.

Marshall W, Gene Therapy Death prompts Review of Adenovirus Vector. *Science* 1999; 286: 2244-2245.

Marshall E, Gene Therapy: Second Child in French Trial Is Found to Have Leukemia. *Science* 2003; 299(5605): 320.

Mauron A & Trevoz J-M, Germ-Line Engineering: A Few European Voices, *Journal of Medicine and Philosophy* 1991; 16: 649-666.

Maynard EM, Visual Prostheses. *Annual Review of Biomedical Engineering* 2001; 3: 145-168.

McCay CM, Crowel MF & Maynard LA, The Effect of Retarded Growth upon the Length of Lifespan and upon The Ultimate Body Size. *The Journal of Nutrition* 1935; 10: 63-79.

McCay CM, Maynard LA, Sperling G & Barnes LL, Retarded Growth, Life Span, Ultimate Body Size and Age Changes in the Albino Rat after feeding Diets Restricted in Calories. *The Journal of Nutrition* 1939; 18(1): 1-13.

McClearn G, Biogerontological Theories. *Experimental Gerontology* 1997; 32(1/2): 3-10.

McKeefery WJ, The Prolongation of Life. *Delaware Medical Journal* 1981; 53(6): 299-304.

McNaughton D, *Moral Vision. An Introduction to Ethics.* Oxford: Blackwell Publishers Ltd., 1988.

Medvedev, An Attempt at a Rational Classification of Theories of Aging. *Biological Review* 1990; 65: 375-398.

Meng L, Ely JJ, Stouffer RL & Wolf DP, Rhesus Monkeys produced by Nuclear Transfer. *Biology of Reproduction* 1997; 57(2): 454-459.

Messer N, Human Cloning and Genetic Manipulation: Some Theological and Ethical Issues. *Studies in Christian Ethics* 1999; 12(2): 1-16.

Meyer MJ & Nelson LJ, Respecting what we destroy. Reflections on Human Embryo Research. *Hastings Center Report* 2001; 31(1): 16-23.

Migliaccio E, Giorgio M, Mele S, Pelicci G, Reboldi P, Pandolfi PP, Lanfrancone L & Pelicci PG, The p66[shc] Adaptor Protein controls Oxidative Stress Response and Life Span in Mammals. *Nature* 1999; 402(November 18): 309-313.

Miller RA, When will the Biology of aging become Useful? Future Landmarks in Biomedical Gerontology. *Journal of the American Geriatrics Society* 1997; 45(10): 1258-1267.

Miller RA, Chrisp C, Jackson AU& Burke D, Marker Loci associated with Life Span in Genetically Heterogeneous Mice. *Journal of Gerontology: Medical Sciences* 1998; 53A(4): M257-M263.

Miller RA, Kleemeier Award Lecture: Are There Genes for Aging? *Journal of Gerontology: Biological Sciences* 1999; 54A(7): B297-B307.

Minuth WW, Strehl R & Schumacher K, *Von der Zellkultur zum Tissue Engineering*. Lengerich: Pabst Science Publishers, 2002.

Miquel J & Fleming J, Theoretical and Experimental Support for an "Oxygen Radical-Mitochondrial Injury" Hypothesis of Cell Aging. *Free Radicals, Aging, and Degenerative Diseases* 1986; 8: 51-74.

Mirandola P della, Oratio de hominis dignitate [1486]. In: Von der Gönna G, (transl. & ed.) *Oratio de hominis dignitate. Rede über die Würde des Menschen*. Stuttgart: Reclam, 1997.

Mizrach S, *Should there be a Limit placed on the Integration of Humans and Computers and Electronic Technology*. Ohne Jahrangabe (http://www.fiu.edu/~mizrachs/cyborg-ethics.html; site visited August 1 2005).

Mooney DJ & Mikos AG, Growing New Organs. *Scientific American* 1999; 280(4): 38-43.

Moore A, Body, heal Thyself. Research on Stem Cells and Therapeutic Cloning: Great Hope tinged With Caution. *EMBO reports* 2001; 2(8): 658-660.

Moore AD, Owning Genetic Information and Gene Enhancement Techniques: Why Privacy and Property Rights may undermine Social Control of the Human Genome. *Bioethics* 2000; 14(2): 97-119.

Morris JZ, Tissenbaum HA & Ruvkun G, A Phosphatidylinositol-3-OH Kinase Family Member regulating Longevity and Diapause in *Caenorhabditis elegans*. *Nature* 1996; 382(August 8): 536-539.

Morus T, De optimo rei publicae statu deque nova insula utopia [1516]. In: Ritter G (Übs. und ed.), *Thomas Morus. Utopia*. Stuttgart: Philipp Reclam jun., 1983.

Moseley R, Commentary: Maintaining the Somatic/ Germ-Line Distinction: Some Ethical Drawbacks. *Journal of Medicine and Philosophy* 1991; 16: 641-647.

Muller HJ, Means and Aims in Human Genetic Betterment. In: Sonneborn TM (ed.), *The Control of Human Heredity and Evolution*. New York: The Macmillan Company, 1965: 100-122.

Munson R & Davis LH, Germ-Line Gene Therapy and the Medical Imperative. *Kennedy Institute of Ethics Journal* 1992; 2(2): 137-158.

Murphy TF, Our Children, Our Selves: The Meaning of Cloning for Gay People. In: Pence GE (ed.), *Flesh of my Flesh. The Ethics of Cloning Humans. A Reader*. Lanham/Boulder/NewYork/Oxford: Rowan & Littlefield Publishers, Inc., 1998: 141-149.

Musgrave DS, Fu FH & Huard J, Gene Therapy and Tissue Engineering in Orthopaedic Surgery. *Journal of the American Academy of Orthopaedic Surgeons* 2002; 10(1): 6-15.

Nadig MN, Development of a Silicon Retinal Implant: Cortical evoked Potentials following Focal Stimulation of the Rabbit Retina with Light and Electricity. *Clinical Neurophysiology* 1999; 110(9): 1545-1553.

Nasseri BA, Ogawa K & Vacanti JP, Tissue Engineering: An Evolving 21st-Century Science to provide Biologic Replacement for Reconstruction and Transplantation. *Surgery* 2001; 130(5): 781-784.

National Bioethics Advisory Commission (NBAC), *Ethical Issues in Human Stem Cell Research (Volume I)*. Rockville, Maryland, 1999.

Naughton G, The Advanced Tissue Science Story. *Scientific American* 1999; 280(4): 60-61.

Nelkin D & Lindee MS, *The DNA Mystique. The Gene as a Cultural Icon*. New York: Freeman and Company, 1995.

Nerem RM, Tissue Engineering: Confronting the Transplantation Crisis. *Proceedings of the Institution of Mechanical Engineers Part H* 2000; 214(1): 95-99.

Nerem RM & Seliktar D, Vascular Tissue Engineering. *Annual Review of Biomedical Engineering* 2001; 3: 225-243.

Nesse RM & Williams GC, *Why We get Sick. The New Science of Darwinian Medicine*. New York: Times Books (Random House), 1994.

NIH Consensus Development Panel on Cochlear Implants in Adults and Children (NIH), Cochlear Implants in Adults and Children. *JAMA* 1995; 274(24): 1955-1961.

Noishiki Y, Dreams for the Future in the Field of In Vivo Tissue Engineering. *Artificial Organs* 2001; 25(3): 159-163.

Nolan K, Commentary: How do we think about the Ethics of Human Germ-Line Genetic Therapy? *Journal of Medicine and Philosophy* 1991; 16: 613-619.

Nordgren A, *Responsible Genetics. The Moral Responsibility of Geneticists for the Consequences of Human Genetics Research*. Dordrecht/Boston/London: Kluwer Academic Publishers, 2001.

Normann RA, Visual Neuroprosthesis — Functional Vision for the Blind. *IEEE Engineering in Medicine and Biology* 1995; January/February: 77-83.

Normann RA, Maynard EM, Guillory KS & Warren DJ, Cortical Implants for the Blind. *IEEE Spectrum* 1996; May: 54-59.

Normann RA, Maynard EM, Rousche PJ & Warren DJ, A Neural Interface for a Cortical Vision Prosthesis. *Vision Research* 1999; 39(15): 2577-2587.

Nuffield Council on Bioethics (NCB), *Stem Cell Therapy: The Ethical Issues. A Discussion Paper*. London: Nuffield Council on Bioethics, 2000 (http://www.nuffieldbioethics.org/stemcells/index.asp; site visited August 1 2005).

Nunes R, Ethical Dimensions of Paediatric Cochlear Implantation, *Theoretical Medicine and Bioethics* 2001; 22: 337-349.

Odorico JS, Kaufman DS & Thomson JA, Multilineage Differentiation from Human Embryonic Stem Cell Lines. *Stem Cells* 2001; 19: 193-204.

Oduncu F, Organtransplantationen. Verteilungsprobleme und Alternativen. *Stimmen der Zeit* 2000; 218(2): 85-98.

Ogg S, Paradis S, Gottlieb S, Patterson GI, Lee L, Tissenbaum HA & Ruvkun G, The Fork Head Transcription Factor DAF-16 transduces Insulin-Like Metabolic and Longevity Signals in *C. elegans*. *Nature* 1997; 389(October 30): 994-999.

Olshansky SJ & Carnes BA, *The Quest for Immortality. Science at the Frontiers of Immortality*. New York/London: W.W. Norton & Company, 2001.

Olshansky SJ, Carnes BA & Butler RN, If Humans were built to Last. *Scientific American* 2001; 284(3): 43-47.

Olshansky SJ, Hayflick L & Carnes BA, The Thruth about Human Aging. A position paper signed by 51 leading scientists in the field of aging research 2002 (http://www.sciam.com/article.cfm?article ID=0004F171-FE1E-1CDF-B4A8809EC588EEDF; site visited August 1 2005).

Orkin SH & Morrison SJ, Stem-Cell Competition. *Nature* 2002; 418(July 4): 25-27.

Orr WC & Sohal RS, Extension of Life-Span by Overexpression of Superoxide Dismutase and Catalase in *Drosophila melanogaster*. *Science* 1996; 263(February 25): 1128-1130.

Panel on the Scientific and Medical Aspects of Human Cloning (PHC), *Scientific and Medical Aspects of Human Reproductive Cloning*. Washington, DC: National Academy Press, 2002 (http://www.nap.edu/books/0309076374/html/; site visited August 1 2005).

Parens E, Is Better always Good? The Enhancement Project. In: Parens E (ed.), *Enhancing Human Traits. Ethical and Societal Implications*. Washington, D.C.: Georgetown University Press, 1998: 1-28.

Parens E, Justice and the Germline. In: Stock G & Campbell J (eds.), *Engineering the Human Germline. An Exploration of the Science and Ethics of altering the Genes We pass to Our Children*. Oxford/New York: Oxford University Press, 2000: 122-124.

Parenteau N, The Organogenesis Story. *Scientific American* 1999; 280(4): 59-60.

Paslack R, Die somatische Gentherapie: technische Optionen zwischen Skepsis und Zuversicht. In: Paslack R & H Stolte (eds.), *Gene, Klone und Organe. Neue Perspektiven der Biomedizin*. Frankfurt am Main: Peter Lang, 1999: 9-40.

Patel NN, Butler PEM, Buttery L, Polak JM & Tolley NS, Tissue Engineering and ENT surgery. *The Journal of Laryngology & Otology* 2002; 116(3): 165-169.

Pedersen RA, Embryonic Stem Cells for Medicine. *Scientific American* 1999; 280(4): 45-49.

Pellegrino ED, Testimony of Edmund D. Pellegrino, M.D.. In: National Bioethics Advisory Commission (NBAC), *Ethical Issues in Human Stem Cell Research (Volume III)*. Rockville, Maryland, 2000: F-1-F-5.

Pence GE, *Who's Afraid of Human Cloning?* Lanham/Boulder/NewYork/ Oxford: Rowan & Littlefield Publishers, Inc., 1998.

Pence GE, Maximize Parental Choice. In: Stock G & Campbell J (eds.), *Engineering the Human Germline. An Exploration of the Science and Ethics of altering the Genes We pass to Our Children.* Oxford/New York: Oxford University Press, 2000: 111-113.

Perry D, Patient's Voices: The Powerful Sound in the Stem Cell Debate. *Science* 2000; 287: 1423.

Peterson JC, *Genetic Turning Points. The Ethics of Human Genetic Intervention.* Grand Rapids (Michigan) & Cambridge (UK): Wm. B. Eerdmans Publishing Co., 2001.

Pierpaoli W, Regelson W & Colman C, *The Melatonin Miracle. Nature's Age-Reversing, Disease-Fighting, Sex-Enhancing Hormone.* New York: Simon and Schuster, 1995.

Polejaeva I et al., Cloned Pigs produced by Nuclear Transfer form Adult Somatic Cells. *Nature* 2000; 407(September 7): 86-90.

Poliwoda S, Keimbahntherapie und Ethik. *Ethik in der Medizin* 1992; 4: 16-26.

Pollok J-M & Vacanti JP, Tissue Engineering. *Seminars in Pediatric Surgery* 1996; 5(3): 191-196.

Pommier JP, Lebeau J, Ducray C & Sabatier L, Chromosomal Instability and Alteration of Telomere Repeat Sequences. *Biochimie* 1995; 77(10): 817-825.

Popper K, *The Open Universe: An Argument for Indeterminism.* London: Hutchinson, 1982.

Prelle K, Embryonale Stammzellen — tiermedizinische Grundlagen und wissenschaftliche Perspektiven in der Humanmedizin. *Zeitschrift für medizinische Ethik* 2001; 47: 227-234.

Proctor RN, *Racial Hygiene. Medicine under the Nazis.* Cambridge (Massachusetts)/ London (England): Harvard University Press, 1988.

Rattan SIS, Gerontogenes: Real or Virtual? *The FASEB Journal* 1995; 9(February): 284-286.

Rattan SIS, Gene Therapy for Ageing: Mission Impossible? *Human Reproduction and Genetic Ethics* 1997; 3: 27-29.

Rattan SIS, Is Gene Therapy for Aging Possible? *Indian Journal of Experimental Biology* 1998; 36: 233-236.

Rattan SIS, Ageing, Gerontogenes, and Hormesis. *Indian Journal of Experimental Biology* 2000a; 38(January): 1-5.

Rattan SIS, Biogerontology: The Next Step. *Annals New York Academy of Sciences* 2000b; 908: 282-290.

Rattan SIS, Applying Hormesis in Aging Research and Therapy. *Belle Newsletter* 2001; 9(3) (http://www.belleonline.com/n2v93.html; site visited August 1 2005).

Rehmann-Sutter C, Why Care About the Ethics of Therapeutic Cloning? *Differentiation* 2002; 69: 179-181.

Reichlin M, The Argument From Potential: A Reappraisal. *Bioethics* 1997; 11: 1-23.

Reinders JS, *De bescherming van het ongeboren leven. Morele en godsdienstige overwegingen bij experimenten met menselijke embryo's.* Baarn: Ten Have, 1993.

Resnik HB & Langer PJ, Human Germline Gene Therapy Reconsidered. *Human Gene Therapy* 2001; 12: 1449-1458.

Resnik HB, Steinkraus HB & Langer PJ, *Human Germline Gene Therapy: Scientific, Moral and Political Issues.* Austin, Texas: R.G. Landes Company, 1999.

Reuzel RPB, *Health Technology Assessment and Interactive Evaluation: Different Perspectives.* Nijmegen: University of Nijmegen Press, 2001.

Reznek L, *The Nature of Disease.* London: Routledge & Kegan Paul, 1987.

Rhyu MS, Telomeres, Telomerase, and Immortality. *Journal of the National Cancer Institute* 1995; 87(12), 884-894.

Richter G & Bacchetta MD, Interventions in the Human Genome: Some Moral and Ethical Considerations. *Journal of Medicine and Philosophy* 1998; 23(3): 303-317.

Richter G & Schmidt KW, Neue Wege der "Gentherapie" — Eine Herausforderung für die Medizinethik? In: Paslack R & Stolte H (eds.), *Gene, Klone und Organe. Neue Perspektiven für die Biomedizin.* Frankfurt am Main: Peter Lang, 1999: 41-93.

Risbud M, Tissue Engineering: Implications in The Treatment of Organ and Tissue Defects. *Biogerontology* 2001; 2(2): 117-125.

Robert L, Aging of the Vascular-Wall and Atherosclerosis. *Experimental Gerontology* 1999; 34: 491-501.

Robert L, Cellular and Molecular Mechanisms of Aging and Age Related Diseases. *Pathology Oncology Research* 2000; 6(1): 3-9.

Robertson JA, Cloning as a Reproductive Right. In: McGee G (ed.), *The Human Cloning Debate.* Berkeley, California: Berkeley Hills Books, 1998: 67-82.

Rohwedel J, Stammzellen — neue Perspektiven für Zell- und Gewebeersatz? *Zeitschrift für medizinische Ethik* 2001; 47: 213-225.

Rose MR, Can Human Aging be postponed? *American Scientific* 1999; 281(December): 68-73.

Rose MR, Aging as a Target for Genetic Engineering. In: Stock G & Campbell J (eds.), *Engineering the Human Germline. An Exploration of the Science and Ethics of altering the Genes We pass to Our Children.* Oxford/New York: Oxford University Press, 2000: 49-56.

Rose MR & Nusbaum TJ, Prospects of postponing Human Aging. *The FASEB Journal* 1994; 8(September): 925-928.

Ross WD, *The Right and the Good*. Oxford: Clarendon Press, 1930.

Rousseau J-J, [1755] Discours sur l'origine et les fondements de l'inégalité parmi les hommes. In: Mairet G (ed.), *Jean-Jacques Rousseau. Discours sur l'origine et les fondements de l'inégalité parmi les hommes*. Paris: Le Livre de Poche, 1996.

Roy I, Philosophical Perspectives. In: McGee G (ed.), *The Human Cloning Debate*. Berkeley, California: Berkeley Hills Books, 1998: 41-66.

Rubenstein DS, Thomasma DC, Schon EA & Zinaman MJ, Germ-Line Therapy to cure Mitochondrial Disease: Protocol and Ethics of *In Vitro* Ovum Nuclear Transplantation. *Cambridge Quarterly of Healthcare Ethics* 1995; 4: 316-339.

Russel DW & Hirata RK, Human Gene Targeting by Viral Vectors. *Nature Genetics* 1998; 18: 325-330.

Rusting RL, Why do we age? *Scientific American* 1992; 276(12): 87-95.

Ruyer R, *L'utopie et les utopies*. Paris: Presses Universitaires de France, 1950.

Salvi M, Shaping Individuality: Human Inheritable Germ Line Modification. *Theoretical Medicine and Bioethics* 2001; 22(6): 527-542.

Sandars NK (ed.), *The Epic of Gilgamesh*. Harmondsworth: Penguin Books, 1972.

Schächter F, Faure-Delanef L, Guénot F, Rouger H, Froguel P, Lesueur-Ginot L & Cohen D, Genetic Associations with Human Longevity at the APOE and ACE Loci. *Nature Genetics* 1994; 6(January 6): 29-32.

Schmuhl HW, *Rassenhygiene, Nationalsozialismus, Euthanasie. Von der Verhütung zur Vernichtung,lebensunwerten Lebens'*, 1890-1945. Göttingen: Vandenhoeck & Ruprecht, 1986.

Schockenhoff E, Die Ethik des Heilens und die Menschenwürde. Moralische Argumente für und wider die embryonale Stammzellforschung. *Zeitschrift für medizinische Ethik* 2001; 47: 235-257.

Schramm FR, The Dolly Case, The Polly Drug, and the Morality of Human Cloning. *Cad. Saúde Pública* 1999; 15(Suppl. 1): 51-64.

Schröder D & Williams G, DNA-Banken und Treuhandschaft. *Ethik in der Medizin* 2002; 14(2): 84-95.

Schroeder-Kurth T, Pro und Contra Keimbahntherapie und Keimbahnmanipulation. Eine Literaturübersicht mit Kommentaren. In: Bender W, Gassen HG, Platzer K & Seehaus B (eds.), *Eingriffe in die menschliche Keimbahn. Naturwissenschaftliche und medizinische Aspekte. Rechtliche und ethische Implikationen*. Münster: Agenda Verlag, 2000, 159-181.

Schwartz WB, *Life Without Disease. The Pursuit of Medical Utopia*. Berkeley, Los Angeles & London: University of California Press, 1998.

Schweizer-Berberich M, Harsch A & Göpel W, Wie menschlich sind elektronische Nasen? *tm -Technisches Messen* 1995; 65(6): 237-249.

Scientific American (SA), Plenty to sniff at. Smaller and More Sensitive Electronic Noses open up New Applications. *ScientificAmerican.Com*, 2001 http://www.sciam.com/article.cfm?articleID=000454C0-FBEC-1C70-84A9809EC588EF21; site visited August 1 2005).

Scully JL & Rehmann-Sutter C, When Norms Normalize: The Case of Genetic "Enhancement". *Human Gene Therapy* 2001; 12(1): 87-95

Seehaus B, Grundlagen der Keimbahntherapie. In: Bender W, Gassen HG, Platzer K & Seehaus B (eds.), *Eingriffe in die menschliche Keimbahn. Naturwissenschaftliche und medizinische Aspekte. Rechtliche und ethische Implikationen.* Münster: agenda Verlag, 2000: 21-29.

Senior K, Germline Gene Transfer During Gene Therapy: Reassessing the Risks. *Molecular Medicine Today* 1999; 5(September): 371.

Shamblott MJ et al, Derivation of Pluripotent Stem Cells from Cultured Human Primordial Germ Cells. *Proceedings of the National Academy of Sciences USA* 1998; 95: 13726-13731.

Shay JW & Wright WE, Hayflick, his Limit, and Cellular ageing. *Nature Reviews Molecular Cell Biology* 2000a; 1: 72-76.

Shay JW & Wright WE, The Use of Telomerized Cells for Tissue Engineering. *Nature Biotechnology* 2000b; 18(1): 22-23.

Shenaq SM & Yuksel E, New Research in Breast Reconstruction. Adipose Tissue Engineering. *Clinics in Plastic Surgery* 2002; 29(1): 111-125.

Shore D, Telomeres — Unsticky Ends. *Science* 1998; 281(September 18): 1818-1819.

Sills ES, Takeuchi T, Rosenwaks Z & Palermo GD, Reprogramming Somatic Cell Differentiation and the Hayflick Limit: Contrasting Two Modern Molecular Bioengineering Aims and their Impact on the Future of Mankind. *Journal of Assisted Reproduction and Genetics* 2001; 18(8): 468-470.

Silver LM, *Remaking Eden. Cloning and Beyond in a Brave New World.* New York: Avon Books, 1997.

Silver LM, Reprogenetics: How Reproductive and Genetic Technologies will be combined to provide New Opportunities for People to reach their Reproductive Goals. In: Stock G & Campbell J (eds.), *Engineering the Human Germline. An Exploration of the Science and Ethics of altering the Genes We pass to Our Children.* Oxford/New York: Oxford University Press, 2000a: 57-71.

Silver LM, Reprogenetics: Third Millennium Speculation. The Consequences for Humanity when Reproductive Biology and Genetics are combined. *EMBO reports* 2000b; 1(5): 375-378.

Simmons FB, Electrical Stimulation of the Auditory Nerve in Man. *Archives of Otolaryngology* 1966; 84(July): 24-76.

Sinclair DA, Mills K & Guarente L, Accelerated aging and Nucleolar Fragmentation in Yeast *sgs1* Mutants. *Science* 1997; 277(August 29): 1313-1316.

Singer P & Dawson K, IVF Technology and the Argument From Potential. In: Singer P, Kuhse H & Buckle S (eds.), *Embryo Experimentation*. Cambridge, New York: Cambridge University Press, 1990: 176-189.

Singer P & Wells D, *Making Babies. The New Science and Ethics of Conception*. New York: Scribner, 1985.

Skalak R, Fox CF & Fung B, Preface. In: Skalak R & Fox CF (eds.), *Tissue Engineering. Proceedings of a Workshop held at Gralibakken, Lake Tahoe, California, February 26-29, 1988*. New York: Alan R. Liss, Inc., 1988: xix-xxi.

Sorg KD, Ethische en juridische aspecten van gentechnologische toepassingen op de mens. In: Prof. Dr. G.A. Lindeboom Instituut (ed.), *De mens en zijn erfgoed. Ethische en maatschappelijke aspecten van de moderne gentechnologie*. Amsterdam: Buijten & Schipperheijn, 1992: 74-92.

Spiegelberg H, Human Dignity: A Challenge to Contemporary Philosophy. In: Gotesky R & Laszlo E (eds.), *Human Dignity. This Century and the Next. An Interdisciplinary Inquiry into Human Rights, Technology, War, and The Ideal Society*. New York, London, Paris: Gordon and Breach, 1970: 39-64.

Stark GB et al., Tissue Engineering — Möglichkeiten und Perspektiven. *Zentralblatt für Chirurgie* 2000a; 125(Suppl. 1): 69-73.

Stark GB et al., Zelltransplantation in der Chirurgie — Realität und Perspektive des Tissue Engineering. *Schweizerische Rundschau für Medizin Praxis. Revue suisse de medecine Praxis* 2000b 26; 89(43): 1737-40.

Steinkamp N & Gordijn B, *Ethik in Klinik und Pflegeeinrichtung — ein Arbeitsbuch* (Second Edition). Neuwied, Köln, München: Hermann Luchterhand Verlag, 2005.

Stephenson J, Green Light for Federally Funded Research on Embryonic Stem Cells. *JAMA* 2000; 284(14): 1773-1774.

Sterkman LG & Riesle J, The Frontier of Substitution Medicine: Integrating Biomaterials and Tissue Engineering. *IEEE Engineering in Medicine and Biology Magazine* 2000; 19(3): 115-117.

Stevenson CL, Ethics and Language. New Haven, Yale University Press, 1944.

Stock G & Campbell J, Introduction. An Evolutionary Perspective. In: Stock G & Campbell J (eds.), *Engineering the Human Germline. An Exploration of the Science and Ethics of altering the Genes We pass to Our Children*. Oxford/New York: Oxford University Press, 2000: 3-6.

Stock UA & Vacanti JP, Tissue Engineering: Current State and Prospects. *Annual Review of Medicine* 2001; 52: 443-451.

Strauss E, Feeling the Future. *Spektrum der Wissenschaft* 1999; Sonderheft 4: 34-37.

Strehl R, Schumacher K, De Vries U & Minuth, WW, Proliferating Cells versus Differentiated Cells in Tissue Engineering. *Tissue Engineering* 2002; 8(1): 37-42.

Suh H, Tissue Restoration, Tissue Engineering and Regenerative Medicine. *Yonsei Medical Journal* 2000; 41(6): 681-684.

Sutton A, The New Genetics: Facts, Fictions and Fears. *Linacre Quarterly* 1995; 62(3): 76-87.

Sykes CJ, *The End of Privacy*. New York: St. Martin's Press, 1999.

Takahashi Y, Kuro-o M & Ishikawa F, Aging Mechanisms. *Proceedings of the National Academy of Sciences USA* 2000; 97(23): 12407-12408.

Takala T, Genetic Ignorance and Reasonable Paternalism. *Theoretical Medicine and Bioethics* 2001; 22: 485-491.

Tännsjö T, Should we change the Human Genome? *Theoretical Medicine and Bioethics* 1993;14: 231-247

Temple MJ, An Ethical Analysis of Gene Therapy as Molecular Surgery. In: Dainiak N (ed.), *The Biology of Hematopoiesis*. New York: Wiley-Liss, Inc., 1990: 347-353.

Terada S, Sato M, Sevy A & Vacanti JP, Tissue Engineering in the Twenty-First Century. *Yonsei Medical Journal* 2000; 41(6): 685-691.

Thomas P, Die neuen Machinenmenschen. *Spektrum der Wissenschaft* 1999; Sonderheft 4: 44-47.

Thomas S, Thoughts on the Ethics of Germline Engineering. In: Stock G & Campbell J (eds.), *Engineering the Human Germline. An Exploration of the Science and Ethics of altering the Genes We pass to Our Children*. Oxford/New York: Oxford University Press, 2000: 101-104.

Thomson JA et al., Embryonic Stem Cell Lines Derived from Human Blastocysts. *Science* 1998; 282: 1145-1147.

Tooley M, *Abortion and Infanticide*. Oxford: Oxford University Press, 1983.

Turner AJ & Coyle A, What does it mean to be a Donor Offspring? The Identity Experiences of Adults conceived by Donor Insemination and the Implications for Counseling and Therapy. *Human Reproduction* 2000; 15(9): 2041-2051.

UNESCO, *Universal Declaration on the Human Genome and Human Rights. Declaration adopted by the Thirty-First General Assembly of UNESCO*. Paris, 1997 (http://www.unesco.org/; site visited August 1 2005).

United Nations, *Long-range World Population Projections: based on the World Population Prospects: The 1998 Revision*. 1998 (http://www.un.org/; site visited August 1 2005).

United Nations, *World Population Prospects: The 2000 Revision — Highlights*. New York: United Nations, 2001 (http://www.un.org/; site visited August 1 2005).

Vacanti CA & Vacanti JP, The Science of Tissue Engineering. *Orthopedic Clinics of North America* 2000; 31(3): 351-356.

Vacanti JP & Langer R, Tissue Engineering: The Design and Fabrication of Living Replacement Devices for Surgical Reconstruction and Transplantation. *Lancet* 1999; 354(Suppl. 1): SI32-3SI4.

Vedder AH, De ontologie van de persoon. Over de morele status van het menselijke embryo. In Brom FWA, van den Bergh BJ & Huibers AK (eds.), *Beleid en ethiek*. Assen: Van Gorcum, 1993: 125-37.

Verzelle M, *Hello Dolly. Kloneren is de toekomst*. Berchem: EPO, 1998.

Viidik A, The Biological Aging is Our Inescapable Fate — But can we modify It? *Zeitschrift für Gerontologie und Geriatrie* 1999; 32: 384-489.

Vijg J, Levensverlenging: de apotheose van de moleculaire biomedische wetenschappen? *Tijdschrift voor Gerontologie en Geriatrie* 1990; 21: 199-204.

Wachter MAM de, Ethical Aspects of Human Germ-Line Gene Therapy. *Bioethics* 1993; 2(3): 166-177.

Wadman M, Germline Gene Therapy ,must be spared Excessive Regulation'. *Nature* 1998: 392(March 26): 317.

Wakayama T et al., Full-term Development of Mice from Enucleated Oocytes Injected with Cumulus Cell Nuclei. *Nature* 1998; 394(July 23): 369-374.

Walters L, The Ethics of Human Gene Therapy. *Nature* 1986; 320(March 20): 225-227.

Walters L, Ethical Issues in Human Gene Therapy. *Journal of Clinical Ethics* 1991; 2: 267-274.

Wang J, Hannon GJ & Beach DH, Risky Immortalization by Telomerase. *Nature* 2000; 405(June 15): 755-756.

Warren MA, *Obligations to Persons and Other Living Things*. Oxford: Clarendon Press, 1997.

Warwick K, Cyborg 1.0. Kevin Warwick outlines his Plan to become One with his Computer. *Wired* 2000; 8(2) (http://www.wired.com/wired/archive/8.02/warwick.html; site visited August 1 2005).

Watt FM & Hogan BLM, Out of Eden: Stem Cells and Their Niches. *Science* 2000; 287: 1427-1430.

Weindruch R, Caloric Restriction and Aging. *Scientific American* 1996; 274(1): 46-52.

Weindruch R, Walford RL, Fligiel S & Guthrie D, The Retardation of Aging by Dietary Restriction: Longevity, Cancer, Immunity and Lifetime Energy Intake. *Journal of Nutrition* 1986; 116: 641-654.

Weingart P, Kroll J & Bayertz K, *Rasse, Blut und Gene. Geschichte der Eugenik und Rassenhygiene in Deutschland*. Frankfurt am Main: Suhrkamp, 1988.

Wert G de, Niet-therapeutische experimenten met (pre-)embryo's. Enige ethische kanttekeningen. *Tijdschrift voor Gezondheidsrecht* 1989; 13(März): 74-85.

Wert G de, *Met het oog op de toekomst. Voortplantingstechnologie, erfelijkheidsonderzoek en ethiek.* Amsterdam: Thela Thesis, 1999.

Wert G de, Humane Embryonale Stamcellen als Heilige Graal. Een ethische reflectie. *Filosofie en praktijk* 2001a; 22(3): 34-56.

Wert G de, Therapeutisch klonen ter discussie. *Nederlands Tijdschrift voor Geneeskunde* 2001b; 145(44): 2109-2111.

Wetenschappelijk Instituut voor het CDA (WICDA), *Genen en grenzen. Een christen-democratische bijdrage aan de discussie over de gentechnologie.* Den Haag: Van Loghum Slaterus, 1991.

Whitaker R, *The End of Privay. How Total Surveillance is becoming a Reality.* New York: The New Press, 1999.

Wick G et al., Diseases of Aging. *Vaccine* 2000; 18: 1567-1583.

Wiestler OD & Brüstle O, Forschung an embryonalen Stammzellen. Was versprechen sich die klinischen Neurowissenschaften davon? In: Oduncu F, Schroth U & Vossenkuhl W (eds.), Stammzellforschung und therapeutisches Klonen, Göttingen: Vandenhoeck & Ruprecht, 2002:68-77.

Willgoos C, FDA Regulation: An Answer to the Questions of Human Cloning and Germline Gene Therapy. *American Journal of Law & Medicine* 2001; 27(1): 101-124.

Wilmut I, Schnieke AE, McWhir J, Kind AJ & Campbell KHS, Viable Offspring Derived from Fetal and Adult Mammalian Cells. *Nature* 1997; 385: 810-813.

Wilner I & Wilner B, Biomaterials integrated with Electronic Elements: En Route to Bioelectronics. *Trends in Biotechnology* 2001; 19(6), 222-230.

Winter SF, Our Societal Obligation for Keeping Human Nature Untouched. In: Stock G & Campbell J (eds.), *Engineering the Human Germline. An Exploration of the Science and Ethics of altering the Genes We pass to Our Children.* Oxford/New York: Oxford University Press, 2000: 113-116.

Witkowski JA, Alexis Carrel and the Mysticism of Tissue Culture. *Medical History* 1979; 23: 279-296.

Witkowski JA, Dr. Carrel's Immortal Cells. *Medical History* 1980; 24: 129-142.

Wolf DP, Meng L, Ouhibi N & Zelinski-Wooten M, Nuclear Transfer in the Rhesus Monkey: Practical and Basic Implications. *Biology of Reproduction* 1999; 60(2): 199-204.

Wolf E, Reprogrammierung durch Zellkerntransfer. In: Oduncu F, Schroth U & Vossenkuhl W (eds.), Stammzellforschung und therapeutisches Klonen, Göttingen: Vandenhoeck & Ruprecht, 2002:55-67.

Wyatt J & Rizzo J, Ocular Implants for the Blind. *IEEE Spectrum* 1996; May: 47-53.

Yang S, Leong KF, Du Z & Chua CK, The Design of Scaffolds for Use in Tissue Engineering. Part I. Traditional factors. *Tissue Engineering* 2001; 7(6): 679-689.

Yang S, Leong KF, Du Z, Chua CK, The Design of Scaffolds for Use in Tissue Engineering. Part II. Rapid Prototyping Techniques. *Tissue Engineering* 2002; 8(1): 1-11.

Yokoyama T et al., Gene Therapy and Tissue Engineering for Urologic Dysfunction: Status and Prospects. *Molecular Urology* 2001; 5(2): 67-70.

Zakian VA, Telomeres: Beginning to understand the End. *Science* 1995; 270(September 8): 1601-1607.

Zant G van & Haan G de, Genetic Control of Lifespan: Studies From Animal Models. *Expert Reviews in Molecular Medicine* 1999; September 28: 1-12.

Zimmerman BK, Human Germ-Line Therapy: The Case for its Development and Use. *Journal of Medicine and Philosophy* 1991; 16: 593-612.

Zimmerman BK, Human Germline Intervention: What's the Fuss About? In: Stock G & Campbell J (eds.), *Engineering the Human Germline. An Exploration of the Science and Ethics of altering the Genes We pass to Our Children*. Oxford/New York: Oxford University Press, 2000: 124-127.

Zimmermann WH et al., Tissue Engineering of a Differentiated Cardiac Muscle Construct. *Circulation Research* 2002; 90(2): 223-30.

Zoloth L, Testimony of Laurie Zoloth, Ph.D.. In: National Bioethics Advisory Commission (NBAC), *Ethical Issues in Human Stem Cell Research (Volume III)*. Rockville, Maryland, 2000: J-1-J-26.

Zuk PA et al., Multilineage Cells from Human Adipose Tissue: Implications for Cell-Based Therapies. *Tissue Engineering* 2001; 7(2): 211-228.

Zwieten M van & Have H ten, Geneticalisering: een nieuw concept. Maatschappelijke verschijnselen in verband gebracht met genetische kennis, *Medisch Contact* 1998; 53(12): 398-400.

PRINTED ON PERMANENT PAPER • IMPRIME SUR PAPIER PERMANENT • GEDRUKT OP DUURZAAM PAPIER - ISO 9706

N.V. PEETERS S.A., WAROTSTRAAT 50, B-3020 HERENT